Glaucoma

Glaucoma

Editor

Rita Dhamankar
MS DOMS
Head
Department of Glaucoma
Laxmi Eye Institute
Navi Mumbai, Maharashtra, India

Foreword

Sushmita Kaushik

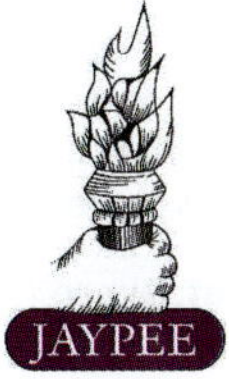

JAYPEE BROTHERS MEDICAL PUBLISHERS
The Health Sciences Publisher
New Delhi | London

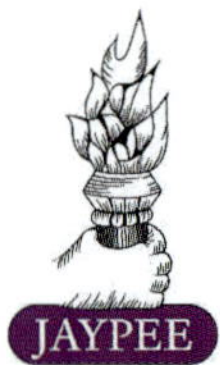

JAYPEE Jaypee Brothers Medical Publishers (P) Ltd.

Headquarters
EMCA House, 23/23-B
Ansari Road, Daryaganj
New Delhi 110 002, India
Landline: +91-11-23272143, +91-11-23272703
+91-11-23282021, +91-11-23245672
e-mail: jaypee@jaypeebrothers.com

Corporate Office
4838/24, Ansari Road, Daryaganj
New Delhi 110 002, India
Phone: +91-11-43574357
Fax: +91-11-43574314
e-mail: jaypee@jaypeebrothers.com

Overseas Office
JP Medical Ltd.
83, Victoria Street, London
SW1H 0HW (UK)
Phone: +44-20 3170 8910
e-mail: info@jpmedpub.com

EU GPSR Authorised Representative
Logos Europe, 9 rue Nicolas Poussin
17000, La Rochelle, France
Phone: +33 (0) 6 67 93 73 78
e-mail: contact@logoseurope.eu

Website: www.jaypeebrothers.com
Website: www.jaypeedigital.com

Glaucoma

First Edition: **2026**

ISBN: 978-93-6616-696-4

Printed at: Samrat Offset Pvt. Ltd.

Dedication

I am indebted to many people who have inspired me to get to where I am today. I want to dedicate this book to the three most important ones.

My husband, Rajiv Dhamankar, who has always stood by me in good and bad times. It was his unwavering support and love that have been my driving force, inspiring me to pursue my dreams with passion.

Dr Suhas Haldipurkar, without whose help I would never have dreamt of coming so far. I thank him for the invaluable opportunities he has provided and for believing in my potential. His guidance has been instrumental in my journey.

Last, but not least, all my patients, who have been my teachers throughout. They have taught me the most through their stories and resilience. Their trust and strength inspire me every day. This book is a humble tribute to all of them.

Contributors

Anchal Gera MS (Ophthalmology)
Senior Resident
Department of Ophthalmology
Glaucoma Services
Advanced Eye Center
PGIMER
Chandigarh, India

Medha Prabhudesai
MBBS DOMS Anterior Segment and Glaucoma Fellowship (Sankara Nethralaya, Chennai)
Medical Director
Glaucoma Consultant
Insight Vision Foundation, Dombivli
Associate Professor
Department of Ophthalmology
Unit of Glaucoma
Bharati Hospital and Medical College
Pune, Maharashtra, India

Meenakshi Y Dhar
MS (Ophthalmology) (Delhi University)
Professor and Head
Department of Ophthalmology
Amrita Institute of
Medical Sciences and
Amrita School of Medicine
Amrita Vishwa Vidyapeetham
Faridabad, Haryana, India

Rajul S Parikh
MS (Ophthalmology)
Medical Director
Department of Ophthalmology
Shreeji Eye Institute and Palak's
Glaucoma Care Centre
Mumbai, Maharashtra, India

Rita Dhamankar MS DOMS
Head
Department of Glaucoma
Laxmi Eye Institute
Navi Mumbai, Maharashtra, India

Roopali Nerlikar
DNB (Ophthalmology) FRCS(Ed)
Senior Consultant
Department of Ophthalmology
Deenanath Mangeshkar Hospital
Pune, Maharashtra, India

Sachin S Dharwadkar
DO (Gold Medal) DNB FRCS (Glasgow)
Director, Samartha Clinic, Mumbai
Consultant
Department of Ophthalmology
PD Hinduja Hospital
Mumbai, Maharashtra, India

Shefali R Parikh
MS (Ophthalmology)
Chairperson
Department of Ophthalmology
Shreeji Eye Institute and Palak's
Glaucoma Care Centre
Mumbai, Maharashtra, India

Shibal Bhartiya MS
Clinical Director, Ophthalmology
Program Director, Community
Outreach and Wellness
Program Director, Marengo Asia
Hospitals
Marengo Asia Hospitals, Gurugram
and Faridabad
Research Collaborator
Department of Ophthalmology
Mayo Clinic
Jacksonville, Florida, USA
Founder, Vision Unlimited
Gurugram, Haryana, India

Sushmita Kaushik MS (Ophthalmology)
Professor
Department of Ophthalmology
Glaucoma Services
Advanced Eye Center
Postgraduate Institute of Medical
Education and Research
Chandigarh, India

Vyshak AS MS (Ophthalmology)
Senior Resident
Department of Ophthalmology
Glaucoma Services
Advanced Eye Center
PGIMER
Chandigarh, India

Foreword

Glaucoma remains one of the leading causes of irreversible blindness worldwide, yet its management continues to evolve at a rapid pace. In the last half-century, the understanding of glaucoma and its treatment has become more variable, complex, and sometimes controversial. Various diagnostic tests have come and gone and are interpreted in many different ways with no consensus on their applicability in clinical practice. Surgical techniques continue to evolve, and indications and value of various surgical procedures also are perplexing. Understandably, practitioners, students, and patients are often bewildered by this battery of information with no common ground.

The current manual is designed to be relevant, scientific, and practical. It has been my pleasure to know the editor of this manual, Rita Dhamankar, for the past 20 years. She is a well-known and respected senior glaucoma expert having trained with Dr G Chandrashekhar at the LV Prasad Eye Institute, Hyderabad, Telangana, India, and Dr Ravi Thomas at the Christian Medical College, Vellore, Tamil Nadu. In 2004, she completed a fellowship training in glaucoma under Dr Paul Palmberg at the Bascom Palmer Eye Institute, Miami, USA.

With this formidable expertise and experience, Dr Dhamankar has accomplished the objective of this book well. The authors have been carefully chosen to share their wisdom as expert practitioners who have explained the pathophysiology of glaucoma and its effective management by creating a sound and scientific understanding of the disease entity. The contributing authors come from many different institutions from across the country reflecting the diversity of presentation and treatment of this complex disease. All chapters are consistently based upon evidence rather than opinions, and where good evidence was lacking, this fact is indicated.

This useful tableside manual aims to serve not only as a comprehensive reference for postgraduate students but also as an indispensable guide for practicing ophthalmologists navigating clinical cases. As the world population ages and the burden of glaucoma increases with dwindling resources, there is a great need for guidelines that concentrate on the essential skills required to care appropriately for the diseased as well as hopefully identify those at the highest risk to prevent them from being visually impaired from glaucoma.

As you progress through the chapters of this manual, we invite you to engage critically with the material, apply the evidence-based guidelines to your clinical practice, and remain open to ongoing learning in this ever-evolving field. Together, through education and collaboration, we can enhance the understanding and management of glaucoma, ultimately improving patient outcomes and preserving vision.

Sushmita Kaushik
MS (Ophthalmology)
Professor
Department of Ophthalmology
Advanced Eye Center
Postgraduate Institute of Medical Education and Research
Chandigarh, India

Preface

To all my Ophthalmologists.

May you never overlook a suspicious nerve.

Glaucoma has been a defining part of my clinical journey—challenging, humbling, and at times frustrating. I have seen patients lose vision not because we lacked treatments, but because the diagnosis came too late, or the subtle signs were missed in the bustle of a busy clinic. Over the years, I have come to realize that while we have extensive resources on glaucoma, what many clinicians need is not more theory, but *a clear, concise, and practical guide*—something that speaks to the realities of day-to-day ophthalmic practice.

This book was born from that need.

It is written with postgraduates and general ophthalmologists in mind—those who juggle packed outpatient clinics, limited investigation time, and real-world patient constraints. It is meant to be a hands on reference, not a dense academia to me, the kind you can flip through between patients or turn to at the end of a puzzling case.

Inside, you will find clinically-oriented chapters, real-world decision trees, annotated images, and practical tips—designed to help you quickly recognize glaucomatous changes, decide when to refer or treat, and monitor effectively. I have included lessons I learned the hard way, cases that made me pause, and shortcuts that actually work.

Whether you are starting out or years into practice, my hope is that this book brings clarity to complexity and helps you diagnose glaucoma earlier, manage it more confidently, and preserve vision in more patients.

Because that, ultimately, is why we all do what we do.

Rita Dhamankar

Contents

CHAPTER 1

Introduction

Rita Dhamankar

Glaucoma is a spectrum of neurodegenerative diseases which starts with apoptosis of the retinal ganglion cells, leading to thinning of the retinal nerve fiber layer and loss of ganglion cell complex. This results in visual field defects, which finally progresses and leads to irreversible blindness. It has some risk factors such as age, rise in intraocular pressure, ocular trauma, use of steroids, myopia, and family history of glaucoma. It presents in various forms, primarily as either an open-angle variety or as a closed angle. It is also sometimes seen to be present at birth in the congenital variety. Secondary causes responsible for glaucoma are ocular trauma/surgery, uveitis, pseudoexfoliation, and neovascularization of the eye. It is the second common cause of irreversible blindness and is known to have very few presenting complaints, hence, it is also called the *silent sneak of sight* **(Figs. 1 and 2)**.

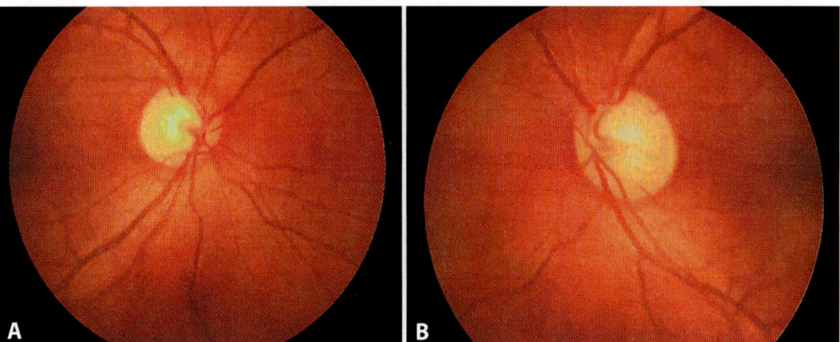

Figs. 1A and B: Fundus pictures in OU showing glaucomatous optic neuropathy showing enlarged cup, thin neuroretinal rims, nasalization of vessels and a superior notch in Figure 1B.

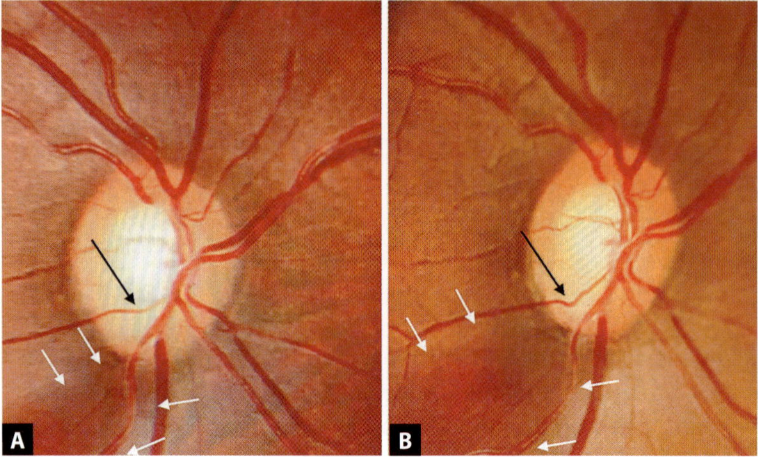

Figs. 2A and B: The black arrows in both the upper figures shows the inferior temporal vessel, you can see the change. The white arrows show the retinal nerve fiber layer (RNFL) defect, which has increased in size, depicting progression.

TYPES OF GLAUCOMA (FLOWCHARTS 1A AND B)

Flowchart 1A: Types of glaucoma based on the angle structures.

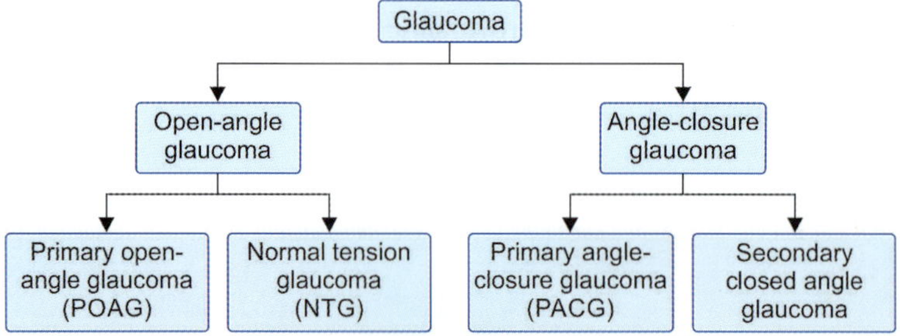

Flowchart 1B: The main characteristics of both POAG and PACG. Also shows PACG to be more common in the Asian population.

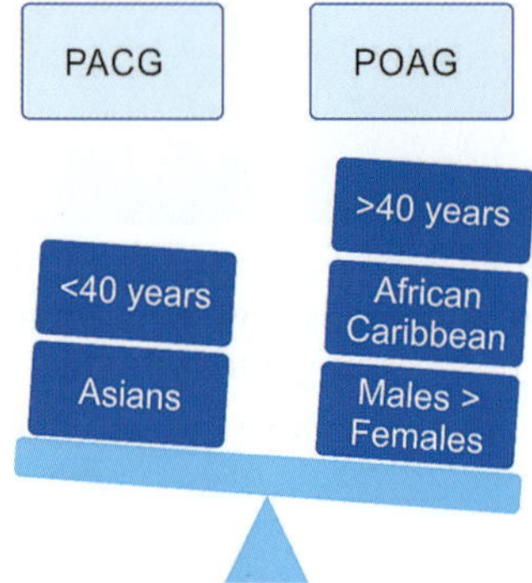

Source: Allison K, Patel D, Alabi O. Epidemiology of glaucoma: the past, present, and predictions for the future. cureus. 2020;12(11):e11686.

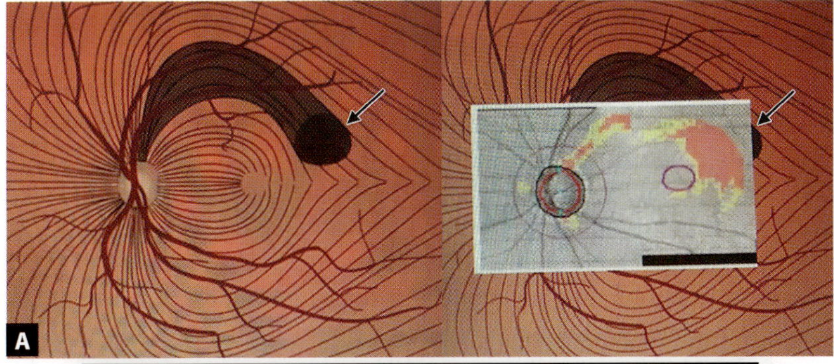

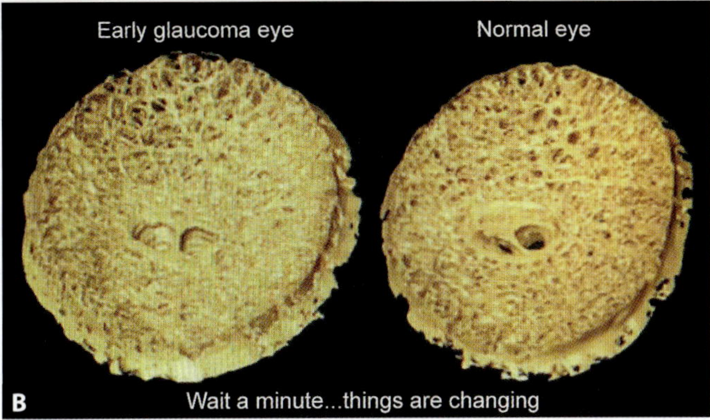

Figs. 3A and B: Glaucoma damages the ganglion cells: (A) The maculopapular bundle being affected in glaucoma depicted in black and on the overlay in yellow and red; (B) How the structure of the lamina cribrosa remodels itself in glaucoma as the affected axons leaving the optic nerve head (ONH).

Source: Roberts MD, Grau V, Grimm J, Reynaud J, Bellezza AJ, Burgoyne CF, et al. Remodeling of the connective tissue microarchitecture of the lamina cribrosa in early experimental glaucoma. Invest Ophthalmol Vis Sci. 2009;50(2):681-90.

PATHOPHYSIOLOGY

The pathophysiology of this disease has been studied over a long period and is said to be associated with both mechanical and vascular processes, due to compression of the axons of the retinal ganglion cells, both due to raised intraocular pressure and reduced ocular vascular perfusion. Various mechanisms like ischemia resulting in hypoxia, chronic oxidative stress, followed by excitotoxicity, mitochondrial dysfunction, neurotrophin deprivation, and mechanical stress probably contribute to the neurodegenerative process in glaucoma. Additionally, cell senescence particularly in the aging retina may also be a key risk factor **(Figs. 3A and B)**.

EPIDEMIOLOGY

Glaucoma is the second leading cause of irreversible but preventable blindness worldwide, and accounts for almost 8% of global blindness.

The burden of glaucoma worldwide was over 60.5 million people in the year 2010 and was estimated to be 80 million by 2020. Out of total of 39.36 million blind people globally, >3 million are blind due to glaucoma. India contributes to the highest (23.5%) regional burden of global blindness. Glaucoma is the third leading cause of blindness in India after cataract and refractive error. In India, the burden of glaucoma is 11.9 million, and the prevalence of blindness is 8.9 million. Glaucoma contributes to 12.8% of blindness in India. It is difficult to estimate the actual burden of the disease and also the various subtypes of glaucoma in the Indian population because of fewer population-based studies and very low awareness and detection rate (over 90% of glaucoma is not diagnosed). Also due to the large geographical and ethnic diversity, the pattern of glaucoma varies in different regions of India. Also, as glaucoma is largely a disease of the aged and we are now seeing longevity in our population, the number of people with glaucoma is increasing at a very rapid pace. So that they do not become an economic or social burden on society, we have to take glaucoma very seriously **(Fig. 4)**.

As it is a silent disease and results in irreversible blindness, if left untreated, glaucoma assumes a place of importance in the health economy of the country. Every patient who is at risk must be examined for the same. At least, all patients who come for an ophthalmic examination must undergo a comprehensive eye examination, which includes a detailed fundus examination, a gonioscopy and a tonometry. A suspect must be subjected to a minimum of perimetry to identify the visual field defects. Adequate chair time has to be spent in explaining the need for a regular treatment and follow-up for the fear of losing sight. Timely and adequate intervention is

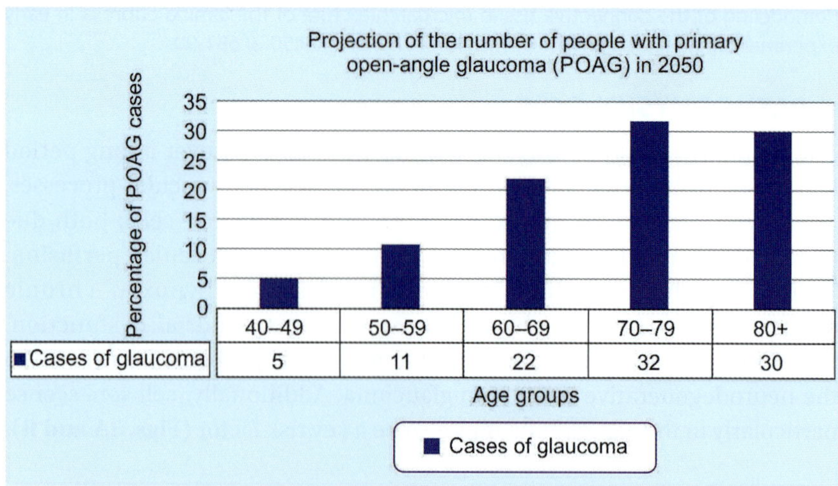

Fig. 4: Number of primary open angle glaucoma in every decade from 40–80+. *Source:* Allison K, Patel D, Alabi O. Epidemiology of glaucoma: the past, present, and predictions for the future. Cureus. 2020;12(11):e11686.

known to prevent progression and therefore reduce the burden of irreversible blindness.

SUGGESTED READING

1. Allison K, Patel D, Alabi O. Epidemiology of glaucoma: the past, present, and predictions for the future. Cureus. 2020;12(11):e11686.
2. Dandona L, Dandona R, Mandal P, Srinivas M, John RK, McCarty CA, et al. Angle-closure glaucoma in an urban population in southern India. The Andhra Pradesh eye disease study. Ophthalmology. 2000;107:1710-6.
3. Dandona L, Dandona R, Srinivas M, Mandal P, John RK, McCarty CA, et al. Open-angle glaucoma in an urban population in southern India: The Andhra Pradesh eye disease study. Ophthalmology. 2000;107:1702-9.
4. George R, Ve RS, Vijaya L. Glaucoma in India: Estimated burden of disease. J Glaucoma. 2010;19:391-7.
5. Jacob A, Thomas R, Koshi S, Braganza A, Muliyil J. Prevalence of primary glaucoma in an urban South Indian population. Indian J Ophthalmol. 1998;46:81-6.
6. Jose R, Rathore AS, Rajshekhar V, Sachdeva S. National Programme for Control of Blindness (NPCB) in the Eleventh (11th) Five-year Plan Period. Community Eye Health J. 2008;21(68):115.
7. Palimkar A, Khandekar R, Venkataraman V. Prevalence and distribution of glaucoma in central India (Glaucoma Survey 2001). Indian J Ophthalmol. 2008;56:57-62.
8. Pascolini D, Mariotti SP. Global estimates of visual impairment: 2010. Br J Ophthalmol. 2012;96:614-8.
9. Quigley HA, Broman AT. The number of people with glaucoma worldwide in 2010 and 2020. Br J Ophthalmol. 2006; 90:262-7.
10. Rao GN, Khanna RC, Athota SM, Rajshekar V, Rani PK. Integrated model of primary and secondary eye care for underserved rural areas: The LV Prasad Eye Institute experience. Indian J Ophthalmol. 2012;60:396-400.
11. World Health Organization. (2012). Global Data on Visual Impairments 2010. [online] Available from https://www.iapb.org/wp-content/uploads/GLOBALDATAFINALforweb.pdf [Last accessed April, 2025].

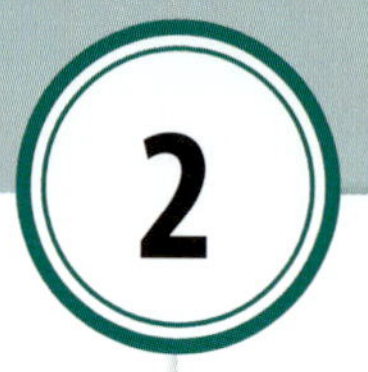

CHAPTER

Diagnostics in Glaucoma

Rita Dhamankar

INTRODUCTION

Glaucoma is a group of ocular disorders caused by multifactorial etiology, resulting in a unique optic neuropathy, with associated loss of the visual fields.

It is known to be the most common cause of *irreversible blindness.*

As it is commonly symptomless and comes on insidiously, it is also known as a *silent thief of sight.*

The only way to prevent blindness due to glaucoma is to diagnose the disease early and start treatment so as to retain all the vision, found at diagnosis.

Which brings us to the point of how do you diagnose glaucoma?

As the disease is virtually symptomless, the onus of diagnosing glaucoma is on the examining ophthalmologist. What all should an ophthalmologist do? There are a few *must* dos to make a diagnosis of glaucoma. Let us look at all of these.

- Good comprehensive examination of the eye.
- Detailed stereoscopic examination of the optic disc
- Gonioscopy
- Tonometry
- Pachymetry
- Visual fields
- Structural imaging of the optic nerve head (ONH)/macula

COMPREHENSIVE EXAMINATION OF THE EYE

This gives one a good idea of some subtle signs of glaucoma may lead to a diagnosis.

- *Size of the eyeball:* A large eyeball in a newborn is seen in buphthalmos, a small eye like nanophthalmos with normal internal structures is associated with secondary glaucoma.
- *Conjunctiva:* A ciliary congestion is seen in an acute angle closure.
  - A conjunctival hyperemia tells you about chronic use of medications
  - A papillary of follicular conjunctiva reveals may be the use of topical steroids in the past.
  - A bleb talks of a previous surgery done for glaucoma
  - A scarred conjunctiva speaks of a trauma/ocular surgery in the past

- *Cornea:* Size of the cornea—small seen in *microcorneas* and large seen in *megalocornea* are both associated with visual disorders.
  - Old *keratic precipitates* means an old uveitis
  - *Corneal scars* are traumatic or dystrophic.
  - *Corneal opacities* can be the result of a corneal ulcer, and may lead to synechiae.
  - *Pigment* on the corneal endothelium can be distributed differently. When in the shape of a spindle, it may be a sign of *pigmentary glaucoma*. Just few pigments spread irregularly could mean a previous attack of *uveitis*.
- *Thickened cornea,* could mean a rise in intraocular pressure (IOP), may be associated with epithelial bullae. It may also be seen in iridocorneal endothelial (ICE) syndrome where the specular examination shows the typical ICE cells on the endothelium.

The thickness of the cornea is an important feature in relation to the anterior chamber (AC) depth, as it gives you a quick estimation of the angle of the AC.

Anterior Chamber

- The depth of the AC is very important. A shallow AC could mean an angle closure. An irregular depth could mean something pushing or pulling the iris. Cells and flare in the AC signifies uveitis. Blood in the AC is traumatic due to neovascularization.
- *Peripheral anterior synechia* due to inflammation, and due to ICE result in angle closure.
- Vitreous in the AC could mean a previous ocular trauma or an ocular surgery resulting in glaucoma.

Iris

- *Absence of iris/aniridia* can lead to glaucoma.
- Vessels visible on the iris/pupillary margin are due to *neovascularization*. Atrophic patches on the iris are telltale signs of an old attack of acute angle-closure glaucoma, typical brown *nodules* are seen in Cogan-Reese syndrome, and *iris cysts/tumors* could compromise the angle, causing an angle closure.
- *Polycoria, corectopia, iris hole formation, ectropion uveae, and iris atrophy* are all common findings in ICE syndrome.

Pupil

- *The light reflex,* both direct and consensual, gives one an insight into the visual pathway, indirectly telling you about the neural status of the eye.
- *Semi-dilated fixed* pupils with iris atrophy are seen in acute angle-closure glaucoma.

- *Loss of pupillary ruff* is a sign of an old attack of angle closure.
- *Pseudoexfoliation* seen at the pupillary margin/anterior lens capsule is associated with *pseudoexfoliation glaucoma* and may also result in a subluxated lens which can result in a secondary angle closure.
- *Sphincter tears* are due to trauma.
- *Posterior synechia* results in buildup of aqueous in the posterior chamber.
- *Lens*: A hypermature cataract, a subluxated/dislocated lens, a traumatic cataract, and a dislocated/misplaced intraocular lens (IOL) can all be reasons for a glaucoma.
- An anterior lens vault, lens protein in a phacolytic glaucoma, and microspherophakia are all associated with glaucoma.

STEREOSCOPIC DILATED EXAMINATION OF THE FUNDUS

The very sight of pathology being the optic disc from where the axons of the retinal ganglion cells leave the eye is what needs to be examined in detail. A detailed chapter on optic disc in glaucoma is included in the book

TONOMETRY

It is the method we use to measure the IOP. What is the IOP? and why is it important to measure it in glaucoma?

The IOP is the pressure in the eye which is caused as a result of the balance of the amount of aqueous that is formed in the eye and the ease at which it leaves the eye.

The Goldmann equation states:

$$Po = (F/C) + Pv$$

Po is the IOP in millimeters of mercury (mm Hg), F is the rate of aqueous formation, C is the facility of outflow, and Pv is the episcleral venous pressure.

What is the normal IOP? Surveys found that only approximately 2% of the population had IOP levels above 21 mm Hg.

This observation led to the belief that IOP measurement above 21 mm Hg is abnormal.

Today many RCT's have proven that IOP is the only modifiable risk factor in glaucoma and hence all of our treatment for glaucoma rests on looking at the IOP. Hence measuring IOP is one of the basic investigations in glaucoma.

The measurement of IOP by a noninvasive device, tonometry, involves applying a force against the cornea that produces a distortion of the globe. There are two techniques, according to the shape of the corneal distortion—indentation tonometry and applanation tonometry. The latter may be performed with a variable force or with a constant force.

The variable force applanation tonometers are Goldmann applanation tonometer (GAT), Draeger applanation tonometer, Perkins applanation tonometer, Mackay-Marg tonometer (MMT), Tono-Pen, and pneumotonometer.

This type of tonometry is based on the Imbert-Fick principle and measures the IOP value based on the force necessary to flatten a fixed area of the cornea. *Goldmann applanation tonometry* remains the *gold standard* for the measurement of IOP, however its use is difficult or unreliable in certain situations where alternative methods have proven their efficacy.

These include:

- In case of nonsitting position of the patient, where Perkins, Draeger, and Tono-Pen are used.
- In case of a corneal pathology, Tono-Pen, MMT, and pneumotonometer are used.
- Excessive lacrimation or poor fixation calls for use of MMT, Tono-Pen, and the pneumotonometer.
- Need to measure scleral rigidity—Schiotz.

Goldmann applanation tonometer **(Fig. 1A)** measures the force necessary to flatten a corneal area of 3.06 mm diameter. At this diameter, the resistance of the cornea to flattening is counterbalanced by the capillary attraction of the tear film meniscus for the tonometer head. The IOP (in mm Hg) equals the flattening force (in grams) multiplied by 10. The tear film of the eye to be examined is stained with fluorescein dye. A split-image prism **(Fig. 1B)** is used to divide the image of the tear meniscus into two semicircles superior and inferior. The IOP is taken when these are aligned such that their inner margins just touch.

Applanation pressures depend on the corneal thickness, as the GAT was calibrated with a corneal thickness of 520 µm. When the corneal thickness is >520 µm, the IOP is overestimated and vice versa. However, there is no standardized correction algorithm for the same. In clinical practice, all you have to look at is that glaucoma in patients with thin corneas is known to progress more rapidly as compared to normal corneas. If, however, the corneas are thick because of edema, the IOP can be falsely recorded to be low.

Other *errors* that can be faced are the amount of fluorescein stain might be too much or too little, giving wrong readings, the patient might squeeze his eyes when recording the IOP, which might give a false higher reading. Astigmatism, corneal scars, etc. can all pose a problem.

The portable version of the applanation tonometer is the *Perkins handheld tonometer*, which can be used in patients, both erect and lying down. Also helpful in camp settings, where there may not be an access to a GAT.

Noncontact Tonometry

Air Puff Tonometer

Noncontact tonometry has gained a lot of popularity in ophthalmic practices over the last few years. It is easily done by a technician in large OPDs. Here, the applanating force is a column of air which is emitted with

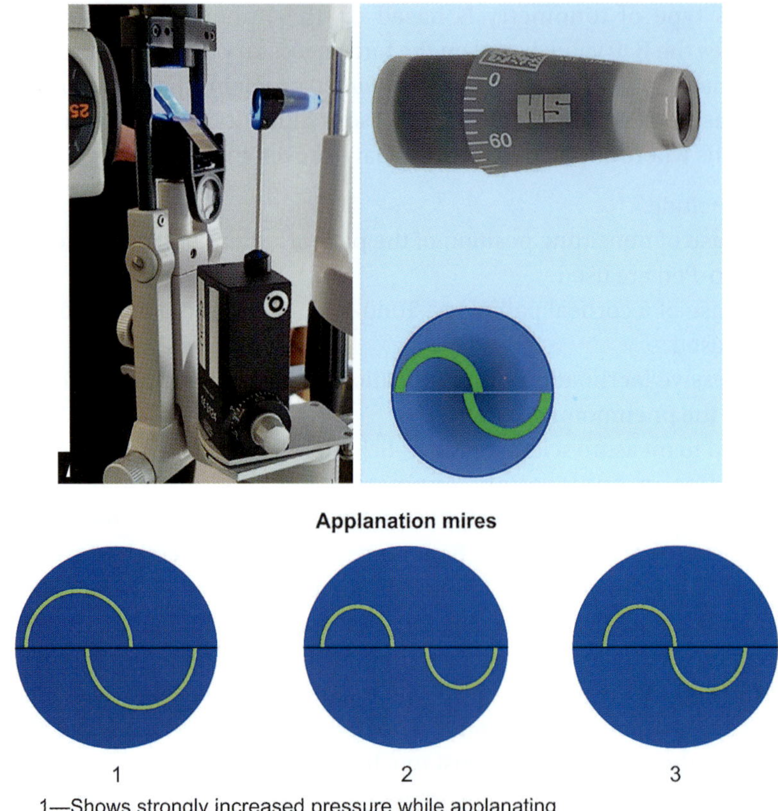

Figs. 1 A to C: (A) Goldmann applanation tonometer (GAT); (B) Prism on the GAT mires as seen on examination; and (C) Misaligned mires, either the mires are too thick, too thin, or pressures cannot be recorded.

gradually increasing intensity. At the point of corneal flattening, this air column is shut off and the force at that moment is recorded and converted into mm Hg. Pressures from these machines underestimate IOP at higher and overestimate IOP at lower ranges as compared to GAT. Hence, it is recommended to take a minimum of three readings which can be averaged to estimate the mean IOP.

Mackay-Marg principle: The tonometer applanates the cornea on contact using a plunger that moves within a sleeve. Applanation of the cornea moves this tip relative to the plunger and this movement is recorded as a continuous tracing following detection by a transducer. As the forces of corneal resistance are transferred to the sleeve, the applanation pressure equals the IOP.

As the area of applanation of the *Tono-Pen* is smaller than GAT (2.36 mm^2 vs. 7.35 mm^2), theoretically the difference between applanating pressure and

IOP is reduced due to reduced corneal resistance of a smaller contact area. The Tono-Pen utilizes microstrain gauge technology and a 1.0-mm diameter transducer tip and is specially designed to fit comfortably in the user's hand, facilitating fast and accurate measurements. The stainless steel probe on the Tono-Pen contains a solid-state strain gauge which converts IOP to an electrical signal. The probe tip is covered by a disposable, protective membrane, the Ocu-Film tip cover. Utilizing a single chip microprocessor, the waveform produced by each touch to the anesthetized corneal surface is analyzed and stored for a statistical comparison process. Leading-edge recognition software ensures that measurements are taken only at applanation, while ScanLock tracking software rapidly scans the electronic measurement data at a rate of 500 samples per second. This advanced microprocessor technology produces objective IOP measurements that are less influenced by operator bias than Goldmann tonometry. The average of four independent readings in case of Tono-Pen XL and 10 independent readings in case of Tono-Pen Avia, combined with a statistical confidence index, ensures accurate, repeatable, and reliable tonometry results. The Tono-Pen Avia has a more ergonomic design, four times longer lasting battery, larger LCD screen, and does not require daily calibration, thus simplifying the measurement process **(Figs. 2A and B)**.

Calibration: The Tono-Pen XL unit is internally calibrated; thus the instrument calibration should be checked only before the first use each day or in the event of unanticipated readings.

The *Tono-Pen*, however, is an important tool for screening purposes, in scarred corneas, through bandage contact lenses and in patients who are unable to sit up. It is an extremely portable and handheld instrument that provides IOP readings that correlate closely with Goldmann tonometry. It is easy to use and operators can take fast and accurate IOP measurement with

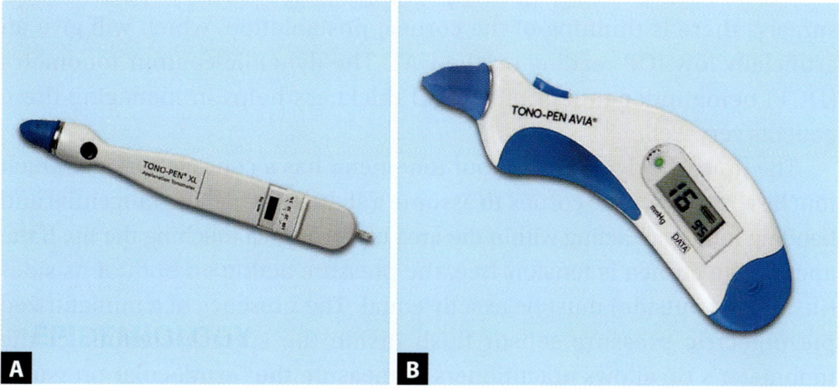

Figs. 2A and B: (A) Tono-Pen XL; (B) Tono-Pen Avia.

minimal training. Moreover, the disposable tip makes the chances of cross infections negligible.

Ocular Response Analyzer: The Ocular Response Analyzer overcomes the problem of corneal thickness. It is a newer noncontact tonometer also using a column of air of increasing intensity as the applanating force. It notes the moment of applanation, but the air column continues to emit with increasing intensity until the cornea is indented. This done the force of the air column decreases once the cornea is indented, the force of the air column decreases until the cornea is once again at a point of applanation The difference in the pressures at the two applanation points is a measure of the *corneal hysteresis*. Mathematical equations can be used to "correct" the applanation point for high or low elasticity. This "corrected" IOP is less dependent on corneal thickness than other forms of applanated pressures.

Indentation Tonometry

The principle of indentation tonometry is that a force or a weight will indent or sink into a soft eye further than into a hard eye. The age-old *Schiotz tonometer* is based on this principle. It consists of a footplate which is placed on the cornea of a patient in the lying down position after the cornea is anesthetized. A weighted plunger attached to the footplate sinks into the cornea in an amount that is indirectly proportional to the pressure in the eye. The plunger sinks into the cornea of a soft eye more than it will into a harder eye. A scale at the top of the plunger gives a reading. A conversion table given with the tonometer converts the scale reading into IOP measured in mm Hg. This disadvantage is due the scleral rigidity.

Dynamic Contour Tonometer

It is very useful in patients who are myopes and have undergone LASIK, as myopes are more at a risk for glaucoma and postrefractive surgery, they may have used steroids for a long time postsurgery. In addition to postrefractive surgery, there is thinning of the cornea, postablation, which will give an artificially low IOP reading on the GAT. The dynamic contour tonometry (DCT) being independent of corneal thickness helps in managing these patients very well.

The tip of the dynamic contour tonometer has a concave surface, which touches but allows the cornea to assume a shape in which no tangential and bending forces are acting within the area of the cornea touching the tip. If the apex of the cornea is tension-free, the pressure acting on both of its sides (inside and outside) must be exactly equal. The presence of a miniaturized piezoelectric pressure sensor flush inside the surface contour of the tonometer's tip allows practitioners to measure the "extraocular pressure" at the corneal apex in order to obtain a direct reading of the IOP at the

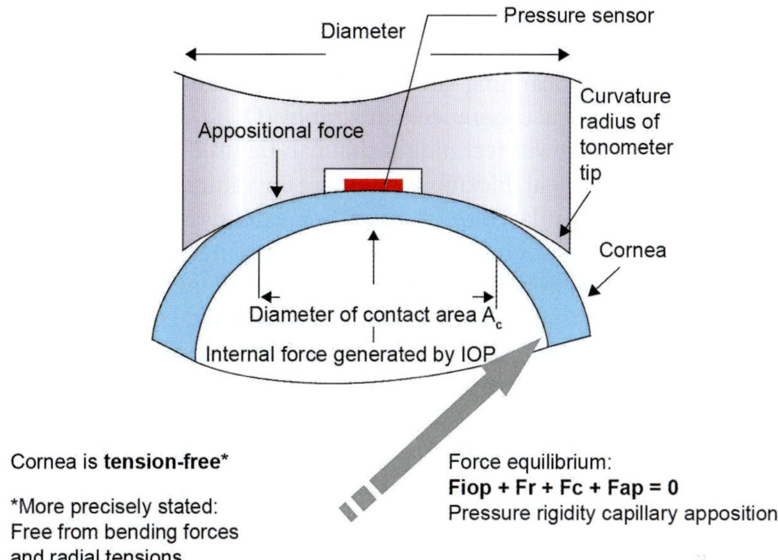

Fig. 3: Displays the principle of the working of a dynamic contour tonometer.

opposite side of the cornea. Contour matching causes the cornea to assume a shape, which leaves it free of any bending forces and radial tension; the pressure is therefore equal on its inside and outside. The pressure sensor placed on the outside of the cornea thus measures a pressure that is equal to IOP. Detailed mechanical analysis by the inventors demonstrated that variations in any corneal properties over a wide range of values does not influence this pressure measurement, and it showed that even the amount of appositional force applied to hold the tip in place does not affect the pressure reading **(Fig. 3)**.

The DCT data were flat across the spectrum of corneal thickness readings, a finding that suggests that this tonometer alone functions independently of corneal thickness.

PACHYMETRY

The importance of looking at the corneal thickness became conspicuous after the results of the *Ocular Hypertension Study (OHTS)* were published. Here, it was found that patients with thinner corneas progressed more rapidly as compared to the patients with thicker corneas. Hence, the revert to the original GAT, calibration which was done for a cornea that was 520 µm thick.

The corneal thickness can be measured by a *pachymeter*. It is a sensitive indicator of endothelial physiology that correlates well with functional measurements. *Optical pachymetry*, which is performed by a device attached to the slit lamp, was found to be not so correct and, hence, is not used any more. *Ultrasonic pachymetry*, which is based on the speed of sound in the normal cornea (1640 m/s), is easy to perform and more accurate. The applanating tip of the pachymeter must be perpendicular to the ocular surface because errors are induced by tilting. Scanning-slit technology, Scheimpflug-based anterior segment imaging, optical coherence tomography (OCT), and high-resolution ultrasonography are newer techniques that can be used to produce precise maps of the entire corneal thickness, including curvature.

The normal (monocular) *human visual field* extends to approximately 60° nasally (toward the nose or inward) from the vertical meridian in each eye, to 107° temporally (away from the nose or outward) from the vertical meridian, and approximately 70° above and 80° below the horizontal meridian.

The binocular visual field is the superimposition of the two monocular fields. In the binocular field, the area left of the vertical meridian is referred to as the left visual field (which is located temporally for the left, and nasally for the right eye); a corresponding definition holds for the right visual field. The four areas delimited by the vertical and horizontal meridian are referred to as upper/lower left/*all the above were structural changes in glaucoma. These structural changes translate into functional changes with loss of retinal ganglion cells. These are documented by testing the visual fields.*

The *visual field* is "that portion of space in which objects are visible at the same moment during steady fixation of the gaze in one direction."

In ophthalmology and neurology, the emphasis is mostly on the structure inside the visual field and it is then considered "the field of functional capacity obtained and recorded by means of perimetry."

A related definition is "the visual field refers to the area visible during stable fixation of the eyes, specified in degrees of visual angle."

A separate chapter has been included in the book on Perimetry and Imaging in Glaucoma

SUGGESTED READING

1. Alimuddin M. Normal intra-ocular pressure. Br J Ophthalmol. 1956;40(6): 366-72.
2. American Academy of Ophthalmology. Basic and Clinical Science Course, Section 10: Glaucoma. Singapore: American Academy of Ophthalmology; 2008.
3. Aulhorn E, Harms H. Visual Perimetry. In: Jameson D, Hurvich LM (Eds). Handbook of Sensory Physiology. Berlin, Heidelberg; Springer; 1972. pp. 102-145.
4. Kanngiesser HE, Nee M, Kniestedt C, Inversini C, Stamper RL. The theoretical foundations of dynamic contour tonometry. Poster presented at: The Annual Meeting of the Association for Research in Vision and Ophthalmology. May 6, 2003; Fort Lauderdale, FL.
5. Stamper RL. A history of intraocular pressure and its measurement. Optom Vis Sci. 2011;88(1):E16-28.
6. Strasburger H, Pöppel E. Visual Field. In: Adelman G, Smith BH (Eds). Encyclopedia of Neuroscience; 3rd edition, on CD-ROM. Amsterdam, New York: Elsevier Science B.V.; 2002.
7. Traquair HM. An Introduction to Clinical Perimetry. London: Henry Kimpton; 1938.

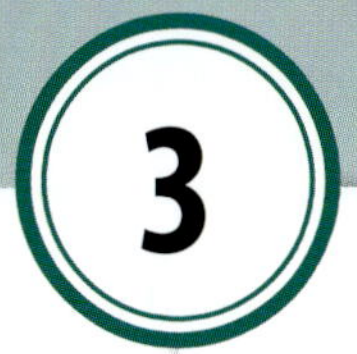

CHAPTER 3

What Role does Intraocular Pressure Play in Glaucoma?

Rita Dhamankar

INTRODUCTION

Many randomized controlled trials (RCTs) have proven the importance of lowering the intraocular pressure (IOP) to prevent the progression of glaucoma. These are Early Manifest Glaucoma Trial (EMGT), Ocular Hypertension Treatment Study (OHTS), Collaborative Initial Glaucoma Treatment Study (CIGTS), Advanced Glaucoma Intervention Study (AGIS), and Normal-Tension Glaucoma Trial (CNTG). It is the most important risk factor and is measured during all examinations without fail. It is the only modifiable factor. It ranges from 12 to 17 mm Hg ± 2 standard deviations in the normal population, skewed a little to the higher side. 21 mm Hg cannot be taken as a cut off **(Fig. 1)**.

HOW DO WE MEASURE THE INTRAOCULAR PRESSURE?

There are many known ways of measuring the IOP. The oldest and crudest of them was the digital method where on applying digital pressure on the closed lids, you could get an assumption of hard/soft the eyeball is. However, that is just a guesstimate and cannot be documented in terms of figures. It is very subjective and varies from observer to observer. However, there are many IOP measuring devices working on different principles which are known as

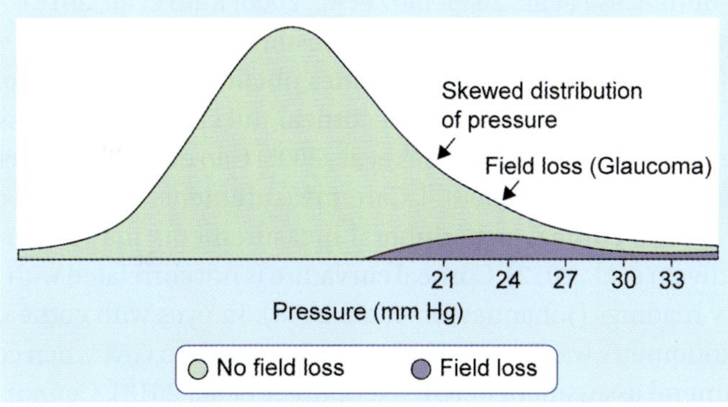

Fig. 1: Skewed distribution of intraocular pressure (IOP) and field loss in a population.

tonometers and can give you a digital value that can be documented from time to time. The gold standard today is the principle of applanation used by the slit lamp mounted *Goldmann applanation tonometer (GAT)*. Applanation tonometry is also used in the handheld, portable *Perkin's tonometer*. The IOP can be measured in the supine position as well, especially in ill patients, or when measuring the diurnal IOP. A good screening tool is the *noncontact tonometer*. Noncontact tonometry offers the benefit of assessment without anesthesia through an automated process with less risk for contamination and corneal injury. Measurements are obtained in seconds and displayed in a digital format. Studies have demonstrated increased utility of the *Tono-Pen* compared with GAT in patients with corneal irregularities such as scarring or in eyes with a history of keratoplasty due to its smaller area of contact with the cornea (Azuara-Blanco et al., 1998; Rootman et al., 1988). In eyes with corneal edema, the Tono-Pen appears more accurate than GAT with intracameral assessment of pressure (Neuburger et al., 2013).

The *dynamic contour tonometer/ocular response analyzer (ORA)* significantly overestimates IOP compared with GAT, particularly at higher IOP levels (Martinez-de-la-Casa et al., 2006). Both Goldmann IOP (IOPg) and corneal compensated IOP (IOPcc) measure significantly higher than GAT with mean differences of 7.2 and 8.3 mm Hg, respectively, suggesting these values are not interchangeable with GAT. Corneal hysteresis was found to be independent of GAT and IOPg but is related to IOPcc; however, studies have shown very small difference between the IOP values generated. The IOPcc in general, correlates with GAT but is less influenced by corneal properties and remains stable after keratorefractive surgery (Pepose et al., 2007). It gives you an IOP measurement independent of the corneal thickness. Then of course is *the transpalpebral rebound tonometer* which can be used without any topical anesthesia in children or in patients allergic to the topical drugs. Rebound tonometry correlates well with GAT within the normal range of IOPs; however, IOP may be overestimated and underestimated at high and low IOPs, respectively (Subramaniam et al., 2021; Fernandes et al., 2005; Martinez-de-la-Casa et al., 2005; Iliev et al., 2006; Kato et al., 2018). At higher IOP, ≥23 mm Hg, rebound tonometry overestimates IOP compared with GAT (Gao et al., 2017). Additionally, IOP values obtained by rebound tonometry are positively correlated with central corneal thickness (CCT), possibly to a greater degree than GAT (Fernandes et al., 2005; Gao et al., 2017; Brusini et al., 2006; Johannesson et al., 2008). I-Care measurements should be obtained from the central cornea, as peripheral measurements may underestimate IOP (Muttuvelu et al., 2012). Corneal curvature is not correlated with rebound tonometry readings (Johannesson et al., 2008). In eyes with corneal edema, rebound tonometry was found to be more accurate than GAT when compared to intracameral assessment of IOP (Neuburger et al., 2013). Cannot forget to mention the age-old *Schiotz*, which has problems with ocular/scleral rigidity, but is a much used tonometer in camps. Last but not to be forgotten is the *digital tonometry*, a misnomer, but come in handy when no other form of tonometry works.

There are *errors in measurements* of the IOP due to many reasons. IOP is dynamic and varies according to the circadian rhythm. It also depends on the CCT as the GAT is calibrated for a CCT of 520 μm. There is no algorithm for correction of the corneal thickness that can be used as a correction factor. It is known from the OHTS study that thinner corneas are known to progress much faster than thicker corneas. Thinner corneas, normally show false lower readings, which could be misleading when treating a patient. In practice due to the diurnal variations in IOP, in real time practice, we are still not sure as to which IOP should we be looking at, the mean IOP, the peak, or the trough. Also, what about short-term and long-term fluctuations? Other factors like breath holding must be avoided when recording a GAT reading. Astigmatism can give wrong readings, 1 mm Hg for every 4 D of astigmatism. The rebound or the transpalpebral tonometer determines the IOP by applanating the bouncing a small plastic-tipped metal corneal contour probe against the attached to a pressure sensor in the tip. This creates an induction current from ocular pulse from which IOP is measured amplitude.

Mires in the applanation tonometry are seen **(Figs. 2A to C and Flowchart 1)**.

ERRORS IN TONOMETRY

Intraocular pressure (IOP) is dynamic. It follows the circadian rhythm, hence, varies according to that. It is very important to note the time that the IOP has been recorded. There can be *measurement errors,* as the mires may be too thick/thin. They may not be matched exactly. We know that the *corneal thickness influences the IOP*. The GAT has been calibrated for a corneal thickness of 520 μm. Thicker corneas record false high readings and vice versa. However, *there is no standardized algorithm* for the same, so cannot be used in real time practice. From the OHTS study we know that patients with thinner corneas are known to progress faster, also patients with thinner corneas give us a false low reading and hence we might be unaware of the severity looking at the IOP in isolation. Herein comes the importance of *measuring the CCT*. IOP as has been documented early follows a circadian rhythm, and hence has *diurnal variations***.** The IOP in the supine position is also higher than in the erect position, so these factors must be noted, e.g., in a patient with hypertension, if he takes a BP lowering medication at night and goes to bed, we are enhancing progression, as he has a low BP and a high IOP when sleeping, which results in low ocular perfusion pressure. This leads to a vascular dysregulation and ischemia to the optic nerve head, leading to progression of glaucoma. To prevent this, the timing of the antihypertensive

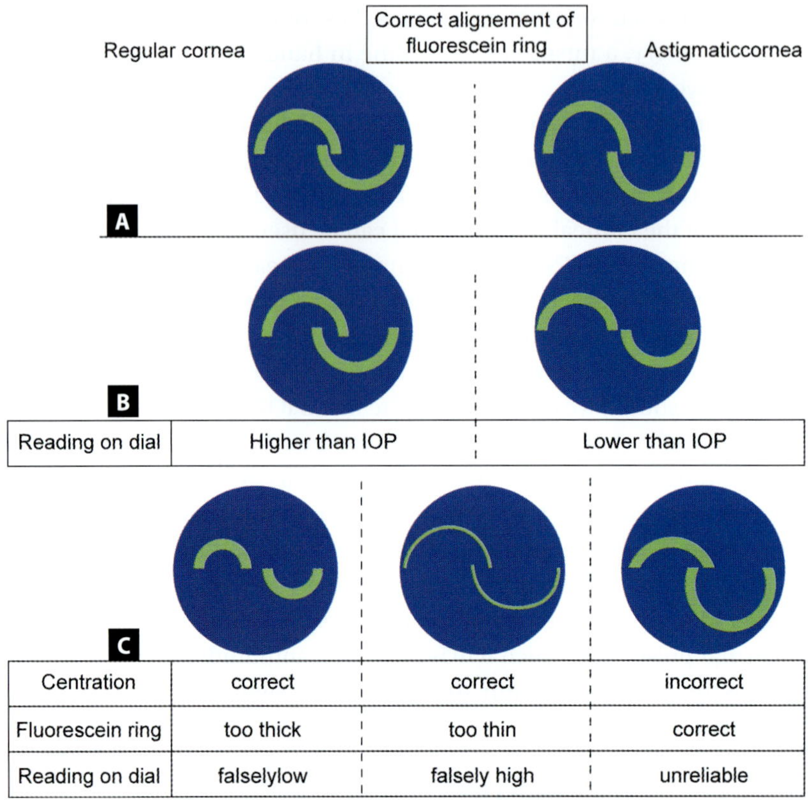

Figs. 2A to C: Various GAT mires interpretation.

Flowchart 1: Classification of tonometry.

- Tonometry
  - Indirect
    - Indentation
    - Applanation
      - Contact
        - Goldmann
        - Perkins
      - Non contact
        - Airpuff
        - Pulse air
  - Direct
    - Manometry

medication can be altered in consultation of the treating physician. As the IOP varies throughout the day, which IOP should we consider in real time? *Should it be the mean IOP/peak IOP/IOP fluctuations? Breath holding* can cause a rise in IOP, and this should be avoided. *Astigmatism* induces a change

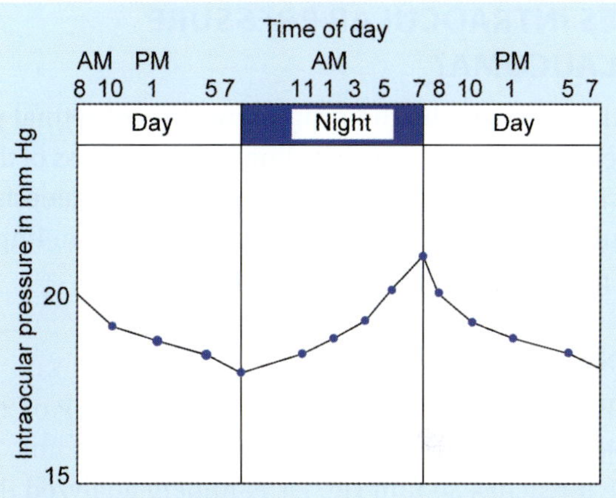

Fig. 3: Diurnal variation in intraocular pressure (IOP).

in IOP measurement. There is a rise of 1 mm Hg for every 4 D of astigmatism. All these factors have a place of concern in practice and must be thought of. We are all aware that we measure only snapshots of IOP which could be changing continuously, there are both short-term fluctuations and long-term fluctuations **(Fig. 3)**.

Diurnal Variation in Intraocular Pressure

Factors affecting IOP: Central corneal thickness, the circadian rhythm where the IOP was lowest between 2 and 4 AM, with a subsequent rise taking place during the latter third of the night's sleep period (Ciulla et al., 2020). Stress changes in body position during exercise and normal daily activities also result in transient IOP changes. Gravity inversion, positioning in the head-down vertical position, can more than double the IOP to pathologic levels, and may even cause glaucoma in circumstances of repeated prolonged activity (Friberg and Weinreb, 1985). In addition to physical activity, use of swimming goggles has been shown to cause IOP elevation by a mean of 4.5 mm Hg, which varied depending on the style of goggle used with one style causing a mean elevation of up to 13.4 mm Hg (Morgan et al., 2008). When changing from the sitting to supine position, IOP increased by around 4 mm Hg in eyes with ocular hypertension (OHT), low tension glaucoma, and controls with no glaucoma risk factors (Yamabayashi et al., 1991). Eyelid squeezing and rubbing can produce large excursions in IOP. Telemetric monitoring of IOP with an IOP implant sensor enabled van den Bosch et al. (van den Bosch et al., 2023) to examine the effects of eyelid muscle action on IOP in 11 patients with primary open-angle glaucoma (POAG). Eyelid rubbing induced an average peak IOP change of 59 mm Hg from baseline, squeezing induced a peak IOP increase of 42.2 mm Hg, relaxed lid closure induced a peak change of 3.8 mm Hg, and voluntary blinking induced a peak change of 11.6 mm Hg.

HOW DOES INTRAOCULAR PRESSURE CAUSE GLAUCOMA?

Glaucoma is characterized by the progressive loss of retinal ganglion cells (RGCs) and their axons with corresponding functional loss of the visual field. While the precise mechanism(s) underlying, the pathogenesis of glaucoma has yet to be fully determined, it is clear that IOP plays an important role in triggering and propagating injury to RGCs **(Fig. 4)**.

When to Treat?

Higher the IOP greater the risk of progression. With IOP of 22–29 mm Hg, there is a 13-fold increase in the risk of converting to glaucoma. This increases to 40-fold once it reaches 30 mm Hg. Dr Palmberg analyzed the AGIS study and proposed the concept of target IOP

WHAT IS TARGET INTRAOCULAR PRESSURE?

The European Glaucoma Society guidelines define target IOP as "an estimate of the mean IOP obtained with treatment that is expected to prevent further glaucomatous damage". The American Academy of Ophthalmology defines target IOP as "a range of IOP adequate to stop progressive pressure-induced injury". The World Glaucoma Association defines it as "an estimate of the

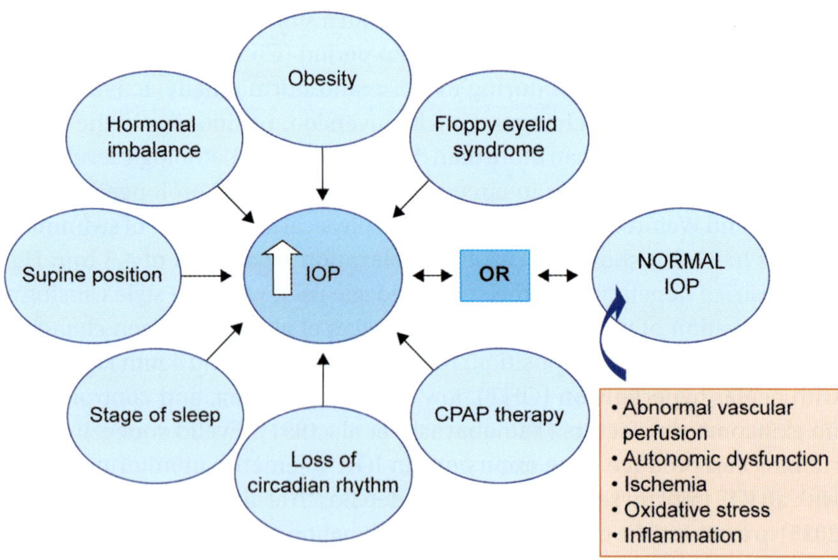

Fig. 4: Factors affecting IOP.
Source: van Gestel A, Webers CA, Severens JL, Beckers HJ, Jansonius NM, Hendrikse F, et al. The long-term outcomes of four alternative treatment strategies for primary open-angle glaucoma. Acta Ophthalmol. 2012;90(1):20-31.

TABLE 1: Recommended intraocular pressure (IOP) range in various stages of glaucoma.

Stage of disease	*Recommend IOP range (mm Hg)*
Early glaucoma	15–17
Moderate glaucoma	12–15
Advanced glaucoma	10–12

Initial recommended target pressure range.

mean IOP at which the risk of decreased vision-related quality of life due to glaucoma exceeds the risk of the treatment".

Notes:

European Glaucoma Society. Terminology and Guidelines for Glaucoma, 3rd edition. Savona, Italy. DOGMA: European Glaucoma Society; 2008.

American Academy of Ophthalmology. Primary Open-Angle Glaucoma Preferred Practice Pattern. San Francisco, CA: American Academy of Ophthalmology; 2010.

World Glaucoma Association Consensus Statement: Intraocular Pressure. The Netherlands: Kluger; 2007.

Setting a "target" IOP range provide an algorithm for management **(Table 1)**. Quality of life may be affected by the medications used. Contrast sensitivity, mobility, night vision, and driving are significantly affected. Attaining a balance is the way to go lowering an IOP to such levels may need medications, lasers, and even surgery in some patients. Should one take a graded approach to get there? A study done by van Gestel et al. proved to the contrary.

WHAT ARE THE MEANS OF LOWERING INTRAOCULAR PRESSURE?

You can lower the IOP by *medications* acting by different mechanisms, reducing the aqueous production, increasing the outflow by both pathways—the conventional and the uveoscleral. You could use *lasers* in angle closure for doing an iridotomy or an iridoplasty, in POAG by doing a selective laser trabeculoplasty (SLT) and, of course, there is always surgery to resort to trabeculectomy, glaucoma valves, or the newly introduced minimally invasive glaucoma surgery (MIGS) **(Fig. 5)**.

Medications

The choice of medical therapy is guided by the baseline intraocular pressure and the desired target pressure, with escalation or combination therapy based on the initial response to treatment **(Flowchart 2)**.

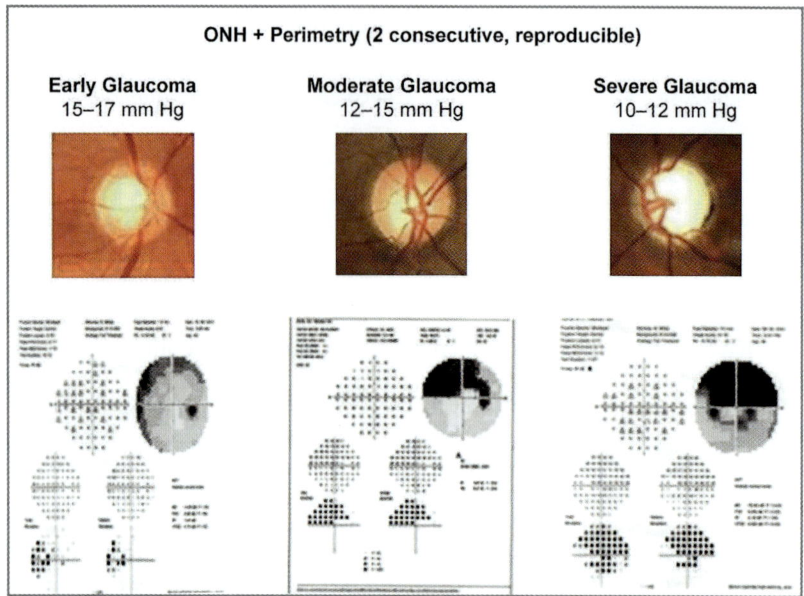

Fig. 5: Clinically applicable target intraocular pressure (IOP) range.

Flowchart 2: Use of medications based on baseline intraocular pressure (IOP).

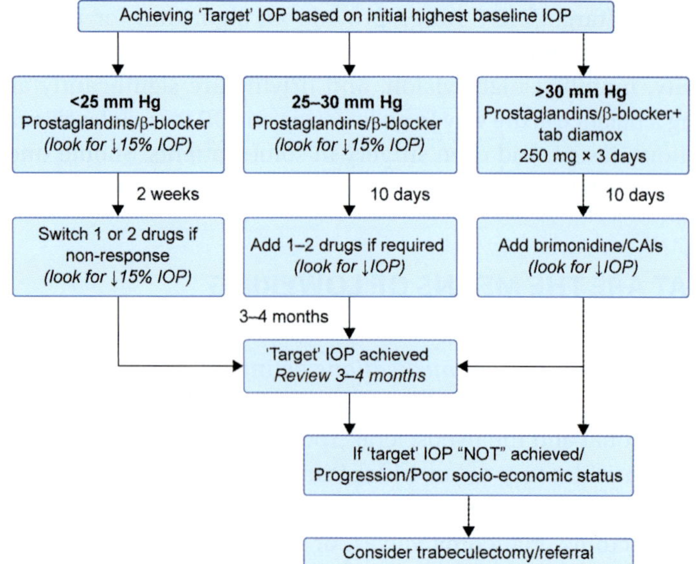

Lasers

Like depicted earlier, a laser iridotomy or a laser iridoplasty is very useful in angle-closure disease as a primary treatment. In the open-angle glaucoma (OAG), an SLT works very well primarily, especially in treatment-naïve

Flowchart 3: Surgical options.

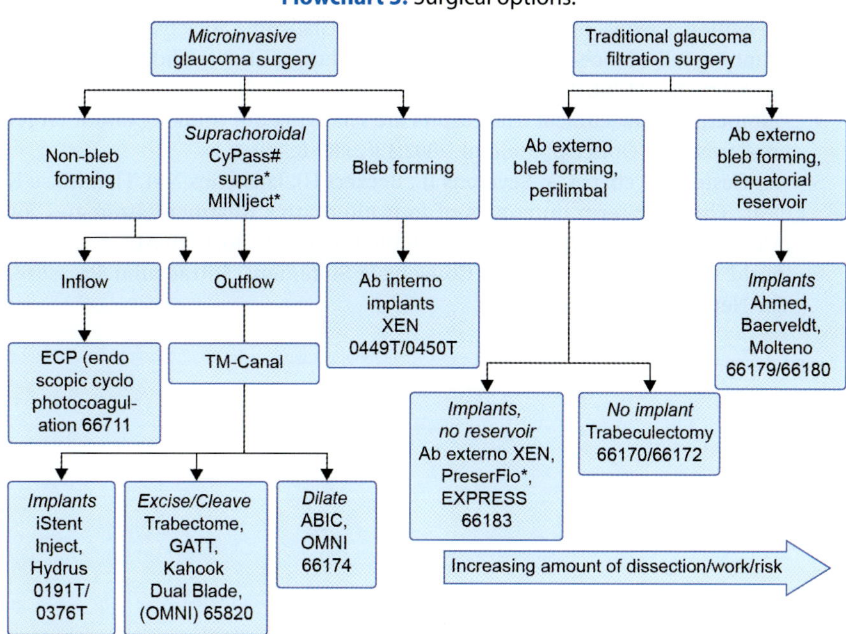

patients. Patients already on prostaglandins need to be kept off prostaglandins at least for a month before SLT to get maximum action. It is a safe and repeatable procedure. The LiGHT trial has shown SLT is a safe treatment for OAG and OHT, providing better long-term disease control than initial drop therapy, with reduced need for incisional glaucoma and cataract surgery over 6 years **(Flowchart 3)**.

What are the Disadvantages of Target Intraocular Pressure?

Once a "target" IOP is set, patients could be stressed if it is not achieved at every visit. There may be possible medicolegal consequences if "target" IOP is considered the standard of care and progression continues. There is no certainty of no progression once a target IOP is reached.

Target IOP is very dynamic. It is possible that the target IOP may be set too low at the beginning. If at the end of aggressive treatment there is no change seen, one may reduce the treatment and let the IOP rise a little to see if the disease stays stable. Vice versa, if the target set is low and more risk factors set in such as hypertension and diabetes need for a systemic steroid for another illness, the target has to be reduced further.

SUGGESTED READING

1. American Academy of Ophthalmology. Primary Open-Angle Glaucoma Preferred Practice Pattern. San Francisco, CA: American Academy of Ophthalmology; 2010.

2. European Glaucoma Society. Terminology and Guidelines for Glaucoma, 3rd edition. Savona, Italy, DOGMA: European Glaucoma Society; 2008.
3. Palmberg P. Evidence-based target pressures: how to choose and achieve them. Int Ophthalmol Clin. 2004;44(2):1-14.
4. Palmberg P. How clinical trial results are changing our thinking about target pressures. Curr Opin Ophthalmol. 2002;13(2):85-8.
5. van Gestel A, Webers CA, Severens JL, Beckers HJ, Jansonius NM, Hendrikse F, et al. The long-term outcomes of four alternative treatment strategies for primary open-angle glaucoma. Acta Ophthalmol. 2012;90(1):20-31.
6. World Glaucoma Association Consensus Statement: Intraocular Pressure. The Netherlands: Kluger; 2007.

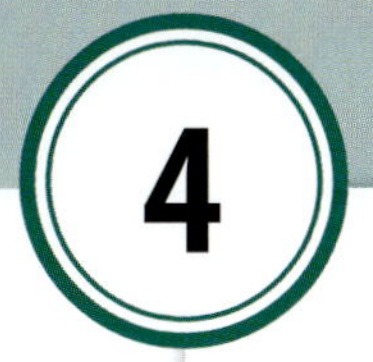

CHAPTER

Optic Nerve Head in Glaucoma

Rita Dhamankar

INTRODUCTION

The real pathology in glaucoma lies in the apoptosis of the retinal ganglion cells (RGCs), which translates into changes in the optic nerve head (ONH). Hence identifying these changes to confirm a diagnosis of glaucoma is very important. In real time, however, both underdiagnosis and overdiagnosis of glaucoma is seen quite frequently.

Let us take an example of a 40-year-old male who comes for a presbyopic correction, he is found to have a large cup/disc ratio (CDR). His intraocular pressures (IOPs) may be 21 mm Hg. Immediately, he is started on an antiglaucoma medication with a diagnosis of primary open-angle glaucoma. His visual fields have neither been tested nor his optic disc size is mentioned. Gonioscopy is a long dream. What if this patient just had a large disc with a large cup? His IOP was just borderline, only one reading, hardly representing what his diurnal pressures would be. No history of (h/o) any risk factors has been looked into, but most people prefer to err on the side of making a positive diagnosis. As against this, there are so many patients who have been regularly under the care of an ophthalmologist, but have missed the diagnosis of glaucoma, as the fundus was not seen/was seen very casually. IOP is only a risk factor, and we know that there is the normal tension glaucoma (NTG) and the ocular hypertension, both of which defy the norm of including IOP in the definition of glaucoma. To make sure, we would do good justice to our patients, knowing the correct features of glaucoma in an optic disc.

What about visual fields for confirmation of functional defects? This is a subjective test, hence, a lot depends on how the person performs the test, also there is misinterpretation of the test, so ideally looking at the ONH should be mastered by all, to prevent irreversible blindness due to glaucoma.

The structure of the optic disc at some point of time in the course of glaucoma is affected. There are many intrapapillary and peripapillary features, in addition to cupping of the optic disc, are associated with glaucoma. Hence a detailed examination of the disc is definitely warranted in screening for glaucoma.

Few features in the optic disc that must be looked at are as follows:

- Optic disc size and shape **(Figs. 1 to 3)**
- Neuroretinal rim (NRR) size, shape, and color **(Fig. 4)**
- Cup/disc ratio in relation to the size of the disc **(Fig. 5)**
- Optic cup shape and depth **(Fig. 6)**
- Optic disc hemorrhages **(Fig. 7)**
- Peripapillary atrophy **(Fig. 8)**
- Retinal nerve fiber layer (RNFL) **(Fig. 9)**
- Presence of disc drusen/optic disc pit

Atypical Glaucoma ONH (Figs. 1 to 3):

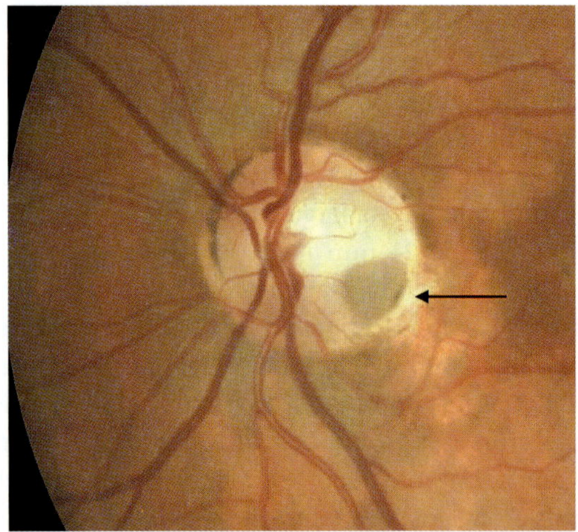

Fig. 1: Optic disc pit.

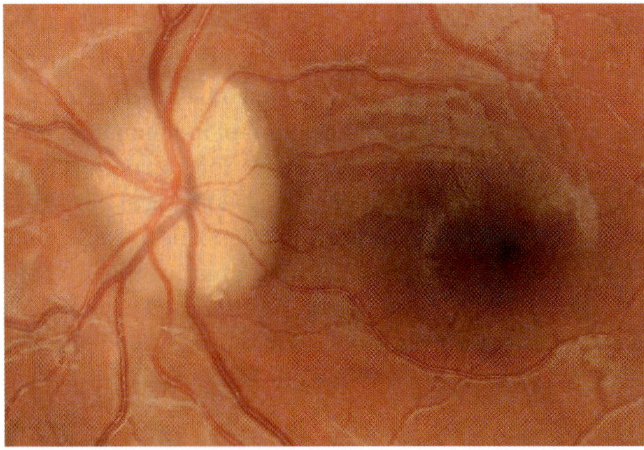

Fig. 2: Optic disc drusen.

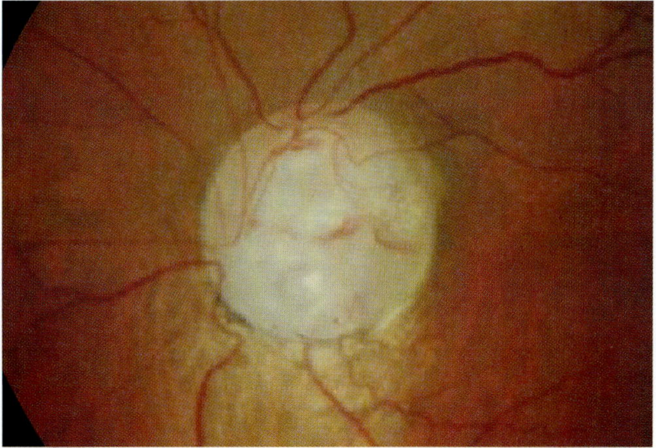

Fig. 3: Optic disc coloboma.

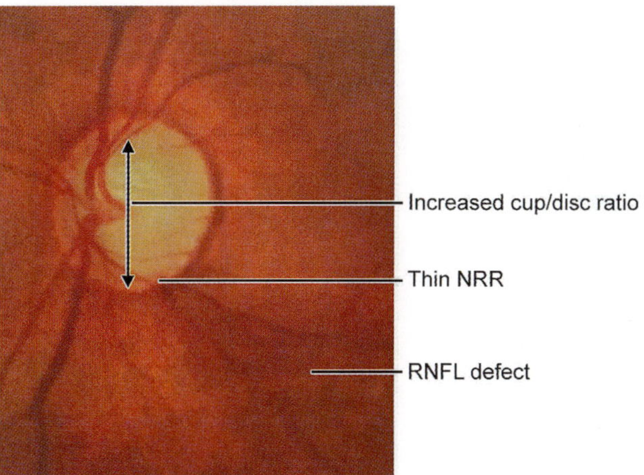

Fig. 4: Features of a typical Glaucomatous disc.

OPTIC DISC SIZE AND SHAPE

The normal disc size varies in people of different origins, but normally the size ranges between 1.70 mm^2 and 3.4 mm^2. Can we determine this in a busy outpatient department (OPD)? Yes, there are two super simple methods: (1) Look at the distance from the temporal disc margin to the macula. It is normally one-and-half times of the disc size. If the disc is large, this distance diminishes, and if it is small, this distance increases. This is a rough estimation, but practically very efficient. (2) The other way is to use a small 5° spot size of a direct ophthalmoscope. The illumination from this spot size should just about cover the normal disc. If the spot leaves some part of the disc uncovered, you can tell that this is a large disc, whereas in a small disc

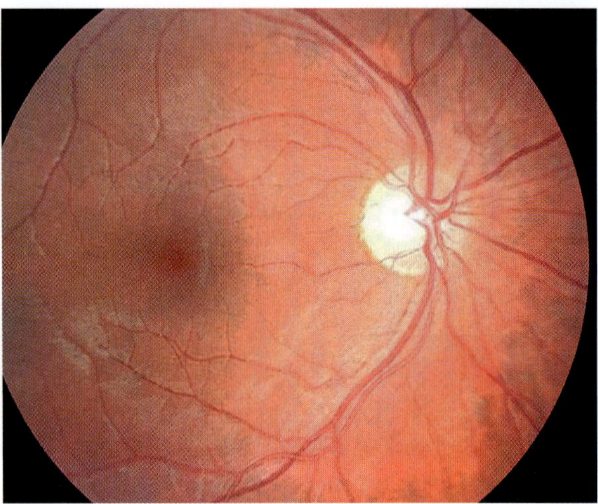

Fig. 5: Neurological optic atrophy how it differs from a glaucomatous disc.

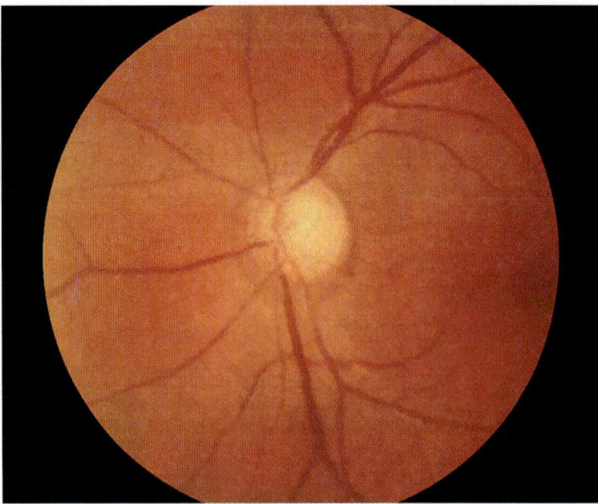

Fig. 6: Glaucomatous optic neuropathy.

the light covers not only the disc, but also some retinal areas beyond it. Large discs are normally associated with high myopia and small ones with high hypermetropia.

The importance of the size of the optic disc cannot be overemphasized in glaucoma. Large discs have a larger neuroretinal rim, hence a larger area over which the nerve fibers can be placed, whereas a small disc has a much lesser area, in which to accommodate the same number of nerve fibers and hence there is crowding.

Small discs are associated with nonarteritic anterior ischemic optic neuropathy (NAION), disc drusen, and pseudopapilledema.

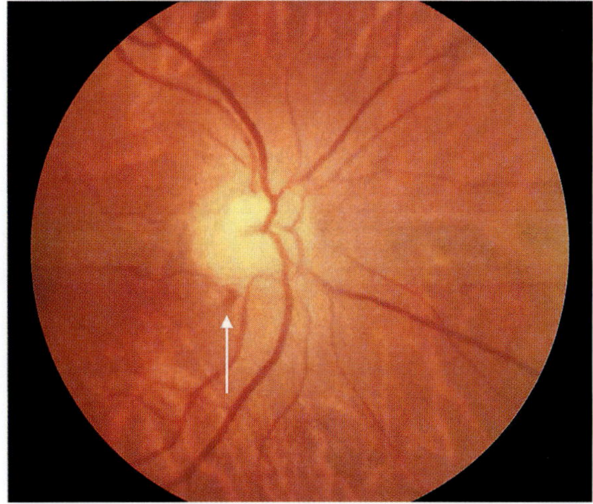

Fig. 7: Disc hemorrhage.

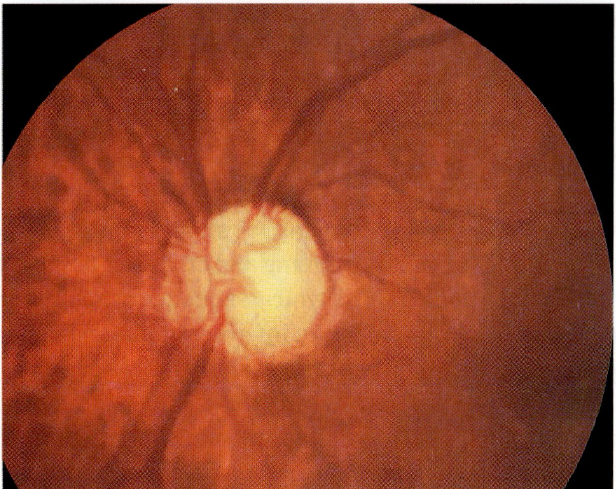

Fig. 8: Peripapillary atrophy.

Small discs are associated with factors that affect perfusion of the disc as seen by greater association with NAION. Nerve fibers are more crowded in a small disc; they are probably more prone to damage due to mechanical fluctuations, also the damage caused to a small portion of the disc involves many nerve fibers fibers; hence, picking up even a small loss in a small disc could result in a larger functional defect.

OPTIC DISC SHAPE

The shape of the optic disc is vertically oval, around 10% more vertical than horizontal. Significant astigmatism could also result in a vertically elongated disc. Those of a highly myopic eye are more oval, elongated and oblique.

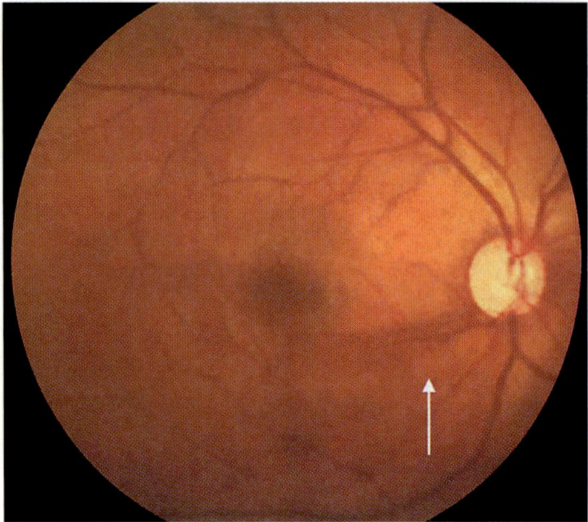

Fig. 9: Retinal nerve fiber layer (RNFL) defect.

NEURORETINAL RIM SIZE AND SHAPE

The neuroretinal rim will reflect selective loss of ganglion cell axons and is the primary location of pathologic changes seen in glaucoma.

The larger the disc size, the larger is the rim area. The shape of the neuroretinal rim follows the ISNT rule, i.e., the inferior rim > superior rim > nasal rim > temporal rim. As clinicians, we should look at the neuroretinal rim carefully and evaluate for any thinning and of the rim tissue, which would indicate glaucomatous damage. The typical sequence of neuroretinal rim loss in glaucoma is loss of rim tissue at the inferotemporal and superotemporal poles, followed by the temporal rim, and lastly by the nasal rim. In glaucoma, these areas are affected differently in various stages of the disease. Early glaucoma usually affects the inferotemporal and superotemporal regions of the disc. As the disease advances, the greatest amount of rim loss is seen in the temporal region horizontally and hence in advanced cases, only the nasal sector of the rim is left. This pattern of rim loss is quite typical of glaucoma and hence it could be useful in differentiating glaucoma from other pathologies.

NEURORETINAL RIM PALLOR

The neuroretinal pallor is often a sign of nonglaucomatous optic neuropathy. The overall disc pallor in advanced glaucoma is more due to the excavated cup rather than the neuroretinal rim. It is often found that the rim may be very thin but pink in glaucoma. Pale neuroretinal rim suggests other etiologies such as ischemia, intracranial growths, congenital, or hereditary optic neuropathies. Pseudopallor may be seen in pseudophakia. In angle-closure glaucoma, where there is a rapid rise in IOP, the disc may appear pale, without much cupping.

CUP/DISC RATIO IN RELATION TO DISC SIZE

This is the one feature that is commonly used by a lot of clinicians to assess glaucoma. CDRs vary even in the normal population. Normally, a CDR of >0.5 is looked at with suspicion, so also an asymmetry between the two eyes of 0.2 is considered pathological. However, a large disc can have a normal/physiological large cup. But, here the horizontal diameter of the cup could be more than the vertical diameter.

Hence, it is equally important to look at the disc size, before jumping to a conclusion of glaucoma on seeing a large cup. Vice versa, it is difficult to see even a significant cupping in a small disc. Early glaucoma may therefore be missed in a patient with small discs.

Hence, this parameter of CDR can be a misleading sign for diagnosing glaucoma if not interpreted in relation to the size of the disc.

The optic cup shape and depth should be assessed based on the contour and not the color. This is very important when the cup is shallow while the optic disc is oriented vertically the cup is oriented horizontally, hence the presence of the ISNT rule. In glaucoma when there is a vertical elongation of the cup, the ISNT rule is broken. Also, in some glaucomas, like traumatic glaucoma with angle recession, juvenile open-angle glaucoma (JOAG) reportedly has very deep cups.

Optic disc hemorrhages are seen in <8% of patients with glaucoma and are commonly seen in NTG. They can also be seen in vascular occlusive diseases, Valsalva maneuvers, and disc drusen. Hence, appearance of a disc hemorrhage is not necessarily diagnostic of glaucoma. But, when seen in a patient of glaucoma is a risk factor for progression of the disease.

PERIPAPILLARY CHORIORETINAL ATROPHY

This is mainly classified into a central β-zone and a peripheral α-zone. While the α-zone is seen commonly in all normal eyes, it is the presence of the β-zone that is likely to be more indicative of glaucoma. The clinical appearance of peripapillary atrophy is a moth-eaten pattern of the retinal pigment epithelium (RPE) temporal to the ONH; if truly associated with glaucoma, there is typically neuroretinal rim thinning adjacent to the area of atrophy. Seen more commonly in myopic discs and tilted discs. The atrophy is generally localized temporally and rarely nasally. These may encircle the entire disc in glaucoma.

RETINAL NERVE FIBER LAYER EVALUATION

The RNFL is a bundle of the axons of the RGCs, together with the Müller cell processes. It can be appreciated best in red-free light. The RNFL is seen as bright fine striations fanning off the optic disc and is most prominent inferotemporally and superotemporally. Healthy RNFL will obscure the details of underlying peripapillary retinal vascular walls; therefore, RNFL loss will present as increased sharpness of vascular walls. Clinical assessment of the RNFL requires a fundus condensing lens, bright light, and a red-free filter at the slit lamp. The green light produced by the filter is absorbed by the RPE and choroid, creating a dark background against which the light that is reflected by the RNFL is well contrasted against the dark background, which allows clinicians easy visualization of the RNFL. Glaucoma causes defects in the RNFL which could be local, diffuse, or a combination of the two. The localized defects are wedge-shaped and are the thinnest at the disc margin and fan other toward the periphery. Notches in the neuroretinal rim, optic disc hemorrhage, and the corresponding RNFL defect are seen 6–8 weeks after the hemorrhage and/or peripapillary atrophy are normally seen in the same sector. Diffuse loss leads to better visibility and hence clearer vessels Baring of the vessels. The degree of RNFL loss correlatescorelates very well to the optic disc damage due to glaucoma, hence, must be evaluated carefully in all glaucoma patients **(Fig. 9)**.

VASCULAR FACTORS

Several vascular changes can be observed in glaucomatous eyes, including optic disc hemorrhages, baring of circumlinear vessels, bayonetting of vessels, nasalization of vessels, optic nerve shunts, and retinal artery attenuation **(Figs. 10 to 12)**.

Baring of circumlinear vessels occurs in areas where neuroretinal rim tissue has been lost, thus the structural support for the vessels leaving the optic nerve is no longer present and is clinically seen as vessels “hanging” across the optic nerve cup without adjacent support of neuroretinal rim. It is a subtle change to look for carefully in order to aid in the diagnosis of

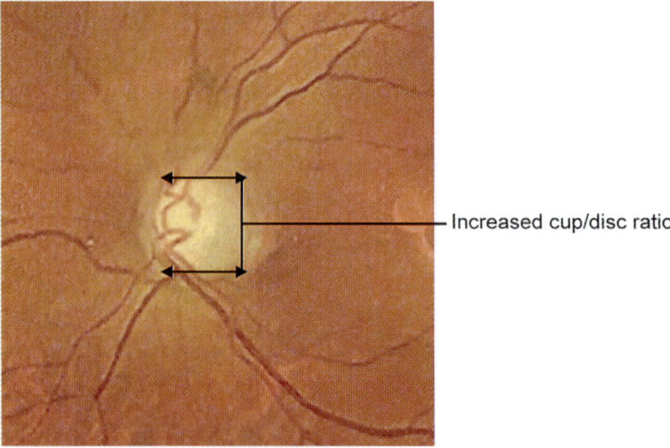

Fig. 10: Glaucomatous optic nerve head with an increased cup disc ration as is shown by the arrow.

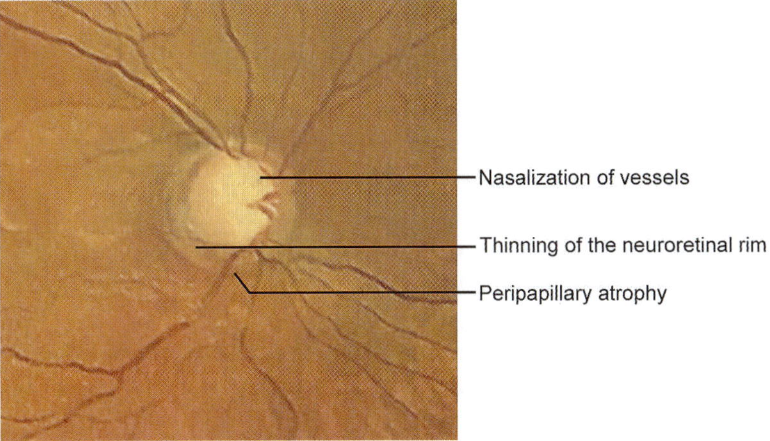

Fig. 11: Glaucomatous disc showing all the features namely, increased cup disc ratio, nasalization of the vessels, thinning of the neuroretinal rims & peripapillary atrophy.

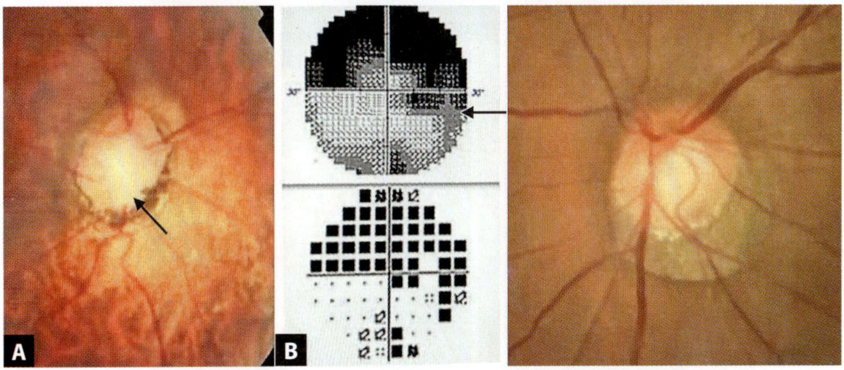

Figs. 12A and B: The same visual field defect, which of them is glaucoma?

glaucoma. Bayonetting of vessels is seen in areas of significant neuroretinal rim tissue loss, whereby visualization of the course of a particular blood vessel is temporarily lost as it makes its way along the excavated nerve borders and reemerges at the edge of the rim from the deeply excavated cup. It is typically seen in advanced cupping or in nerves with localized notching of the neuroretinal rim. Nasalization of blood vessels occurs in very advanced glaucoma whereby the only structural support remains along the nasal rim due to severe loss of superior, inferior, and temporal rim tissue. It is easily observable in advanced cupping and will not be present in early disease. Retinal artery attenuation can also occur in glaucomatous eyes, but is typically a subtler finding than the aforementioned vascular changes. It likely results due to decreased metabolic demand from an increasingly thinner rim tissue. It is a very subtle but important change to look for in helping the clinician determine the level of suspicion for early glaucoma.

TYPICAL GLAUCOMA DISC

Signs of glaucoma in the optic nerve head:

The 5R rule can be applied to identify a glaucomatous disc:

1. Scleral RING to estimate the size of the disc **(Figs. 13A and B)**
2. Neuroretinal RIM to look at the area of the rim
3. RNFL defects in the RNFL layer
4. Peripapillary Region. β-zone
5. Retinal and optic disc hemorrhages
    - Generalized/focal enlargement of the cup
    - Disc hemorrhage (within 1 disc diameter of ONH) **(Figs. 14A and B)**
    - Thinning of neuroretinal rim (usually at superior and inferior poles) ISNT rule

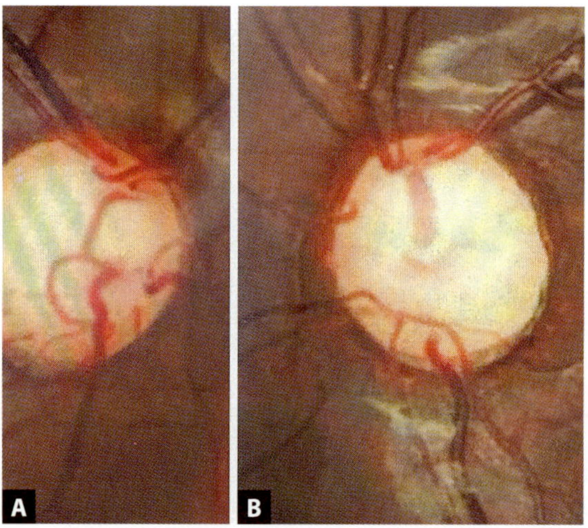

Figs. 13A and B: Do discs shown in **Figures 12A and B** depict glaucoma?

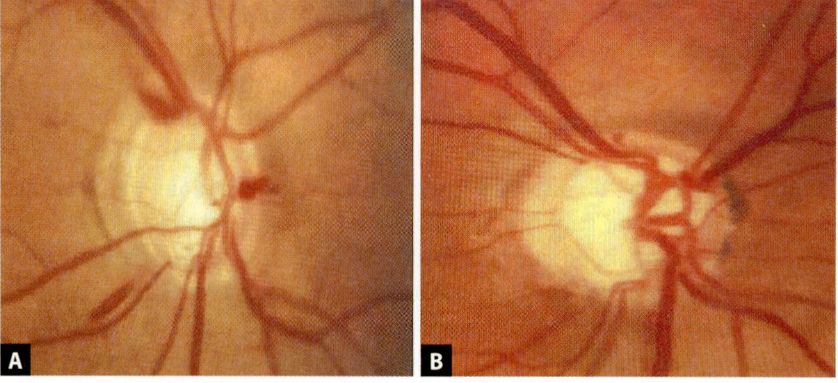

Figs. 14A and B: What signs of glaucoma can you *see* in **Figures 14A and B**? What does it signify?

- Asymmetry of cupping between patient's eyes >0.2
- Loss of nerve fiber layer
- Parapapillary atrophy β-zone parapapillary atrophy (more common in glaucomatous eyes)
- The ONH can be estimated by the direct ophthalmoscope, the indirect ophthalmoscope, or with the help of the coaxial illumination of the slit lamp using a condensing lens 60/78/90 Diopters. The last being the best, as it gives you a good stereoscopic view of the disc.

The strategy to examine the ONH:

- Dilate pupils, if possible and safe to do so
- Identify disc edge and cup edge thereby identifying rim
- Does the rim thickness obey the ISNT rule?
- Is there a hemorrhage?
- Estimate vertical CDR
- Measure size of ONH
- Examine the retinal nerve fiber layer (using green light)

How do you identify the disc size clinically? A simple method is to estimate the number of discs that you can place from the temporal margin of the disc to the macula. In normal eyes, the distance between the disc and center of the fovea is approximately 2.5 disc diameters, as measured from the temporal edge of the disc to the center of the fovea. If you have a large disc you cannot fit this, as the area occupied by one you can easily fit three discs or more.

Why is it important to know the disc size, is that, the large disc may have a normally large cup as against small discs where there are the number of RCG'S is concentrated in the place and hereon. In case of atrophy of these axons, the cup enlarges, hence even a small enlargement of the cup in a small disc means a lot more loss of axons as compared to a large-sized disc. In normal eyes, the distance between the disc and center of the fovea is approximately *2.5–3 disc diameters,* as measured from the temporal edge of the disc to the center of the fovea **(Figs. 15A and B)**.

Normally, the neuroretinal rim follows the ISNT rule, which states that the inferior rim > superior rim > nasal rim > temporal rim. If this ratio is not followed, suspect a damage to the neuroretinal rim which could be glaucomatous.

Disc hemorrhages within 1 disc diameter is a precursor of loss of the RNFL. Look for it carefully. Many times a disc photograph shows up a hemorrhages even before being picked up on manual examination.

A RNFL loss is easily picked up on a red-free examination as a dark wedge, as shown in the photograph.

Beta-zone atrophy in the parapapillary is normally seen in glaucoma.

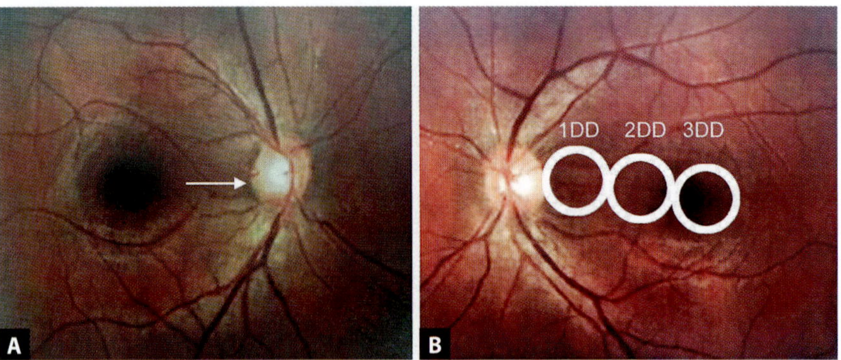

Figs. 15A and B: Normal disc where 2.5 discs fit from the temporal margin of the disc to the center of the fovea.

Always make sure to draw an annotated diagram of the ONH/if possible, take a fundus photograph for documentation.

PEARLS OF A GLAUCOMATOUS OPTIC NERVE HEAD

- Excavation of the neuroretinal rim is a definite sign of glaucomatous optic neuropathy, as is loss of the ISNT rule.
- Pallor of the optic disc may be seen in advanced glaucoma; however, disc pallor should raise a suspicion of a different pathology like an optic atrophy.
- A color cup does not necessarily identify the edge of the cup. The contour cup identified by change in the direction of the blood vessels is a more reliable way to identify the edge of the cup.
- *Always corelate the disc findings with the visual field defect.* Where this is not the case, further investigations (e.g., CT/MRI scan) may be indicated.
- The size of the cup always appears smaller when viewed monoscopically, hence a stereoscopic view is a must. So also, the cup edge can be identified very well on a stereoscopic view.
- A measurement of CDR alone is inadequate in diagnosing glaucoma, as explained earlier. Large discs can have large discs which could be normal and small discs will have smaller cups and hence a smaller CDR.
- Loss of RNFL, disc hemorrhages, and the presence of a peripapillary atrophy are findings to be also looked for.

SUGGESTED READING

1. Arvind H, George R, Raju P, Ve RS, Mani B, Kannan P, Vijaya L. Neural rim characteristics of healthy South Indians: the Chennai Glaucoma Study. Invest Ophthalmol Vis Sci. 2008 Aug;49(8):3457–3464. doi: 10.1167/iovs.07-1210

2. Jonas JB, Gusek GC, Naumann GO. Optic disc, cup and neuroretinal rim size, configuration and correlations in normal eyes. Invest Ophthalmol Vis Sci. 1988;29(7):1151-8.
3. Jonas JB, Schiro D. Localised wedge shaped defects of the retinal nerve fibre layer in glaucoma. Br J Ophthalmol. 1994;78(4):285-90.
4. Jonas JB, Thomas R, George R, Berenshtein E, Muliyil J. Optic disc morphology in south India: the Vellore Eye Study. Br J Ophthalmol. 2003;87(2):189-96.
5. Sekhar GC, Prasad K, Dandona R, John RK, Dandona L. Planimetric optic disc parameters in normal eyes: a population-based study in South India. Indian J Ophthalmol. 2001;49(1):19-23.

CHAPTER

Perimetry

Rita Dhamankar

INTRODUCTION

The measurement of visual functions of the eye at topographically defined loci in the visual field is called perimetry. There are a few terminologies that we need to know when interpreting a perimetry printout.

- *Threshold:* A given stimulus is seen 50% and missed 50% of times.
- *Suprathreshold:* 95% chance of a stimulus is seen.
- *Infrathreshold:* <5% chance of a stimulus is seen.
- *Isopter:* Border that connects the threshold points of a given stimulus

  Perimetry is done in two ways: (1) static perimetry and (2) kinetic perimetry.

KINETIC PERIMETRY

It uses a moving illuminated target and is done manually (e.g., Goldmann). Stimulus is moved from a nonseeing area of visual field to a seeing area along a set meridian and other meridians which are usually 15° apart.

Luminance and size of target: Changed to plot areas of different light sensitivities

The advantages of kinetic perimetry are as follows:

- Moving targets can define isopter contours and scotomas rapidly
- It is relatively inexpensive and durable
- Patients are comfortable.

The *disadvantages of kinetic perimetry* are as follows:

- Technical skills, training, and retraining personnel are a must.
- Early or subtle changes can be overlooked.
- Statistical analysis is difficult.

STATIC PERIMETRY

It is a computerized perimetry where the stimulus is constant and the brightness varies. Here, the Z-axis or the hill of vision is also mapped.

The *advantages of the static perimetry* are as follows:

- The data are quantifiable, reproducible, and amenable to statistical manipulation.
- Threshold detection is more sensitive.
- Reduced need for highly trained technicians

Disadvantages of the static perimetry: The instrument is very expensive. The amount of data generated is huge. It can be very difficult to interpret the data, unless you are trained to interpret it systematically.

The current gold standard of testing is the static or automated perimetry. It has reproducible testing conditions. It has huge data storage capability, has more sensitive testing, and is very easy to learn and use.

What is it that we need to know from perimetry?

- To identify a defect on the visual field
- To, then, see if the defect is glaucomatous.
- To check out if it is stable or progressing.
- To look at the extent/depth of the defect/look for a new defect

How is perimetry done? The patient looks into a white hemispherical bowl at a small fixation point at the center. At fixed stationary locations the visual field stimuli are briefly presented usually for about 200 milliseconds duration. The patient presses a response button when the stimulus is detected. The stimulus is affected by the size, its brightness, and the background illumination. Of these, only the stimulus brightness varies whereas the stimulus size and the background illumination is constant.

STIMULUS SIZE

The size of the stimulus used in perimetry plays an important role in determining retinal sensitivity. In routine clinical practice, Goldmann stimulus sizes are commonly used. These stimuli vary in diameter and area and are designated from size 0 to size V. The diameter and area of the different Goldmann stimulus sizes are summarized in **Table 1**.

TABLE 1: Size of Goldmann targets.

Goldmann stimulus size	*Diameter (mm)*	*Area (mm^2)*
0	0.28	1/16
I	0.56	¼
II	1.13	1
III	2.26	4
IV	4.51	16
V	9.03	64

Background illlumination differs for every machine.

For the Humphrey perimeter it is: 31.5 apostilbs (asb) (10 cd/m^2), where apostilbs: absolute measure of luminance and 1 apostilbs: 0.3183 candela/m^2.

The stimulus intensity is varied by the use of attenuation filters. The attenuation of light is expressed in logarithmic units. 1 decibel = 1/10 log unit of attenuation of maximum available stimulus. 10,000 asb units is used for the current Humphrey perimeters. Being a log unit, as the intensity increases the decibel value of light decreases. The brighter the stimulus the lower is the

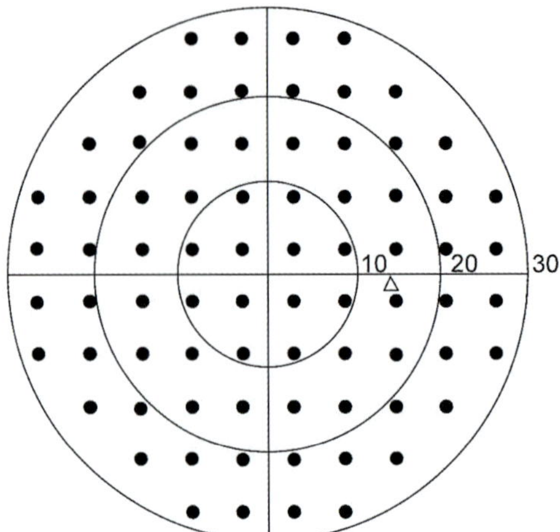

Fig. 1: Displaying the points tested on a 30-2 program on a Humphrey visual field (HVF).

threshold, lower the dB, and vice versa. Closer to the fovea, the dB value is higher than at the periphery.

Testing strategy: It differs with every machine. We shall take the Humphrey machine as our standard and discuss the various strategies used for testing glaucoma in a Humphrey machine.

To detect glaucoma field defects according to the stage of glaucoma.

The 30-2 central threshold test pattern where number of test points is 76. There is a bare area of 3° which is left surrounding the fixation spot. The points are spread in 3° area from fixation point. The distance between two points is 6° (the point density is 6°) as shown in the **Figure 1**.

24-2 central threshold test pattern: In the 24-2, the number of test points is 54.

The four innermost points are 3° from the fixation spot. An area of 3° is left surrounding the fixation spot. The distance between each two points is 6° **(Fig. 2)**.

10-2 central threshold test pattern: The number of test points in this program is 68. The four innermost points are 1° from the fixation spot. A bare area of 1° is left surrounding the fixation spot. The distance between each two points is 2°. This test helps to see an enlarged area around the macula, which affects the visual function most **(Fig. 3)**.

Macular programming test pattern: The number of tested points is 16. The two innermost points are 1° from the fixation spot. A 1° of bare area is left surrounding the fixation spot. The distance between each two points is 2° **(Fig. 4)**.

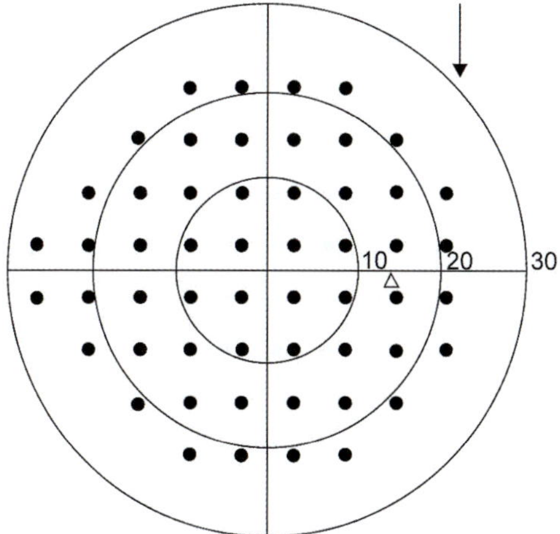

Fig. 2: Displaying the points tested on a 24-2 program. Note the inclusion of two extra nasal points.

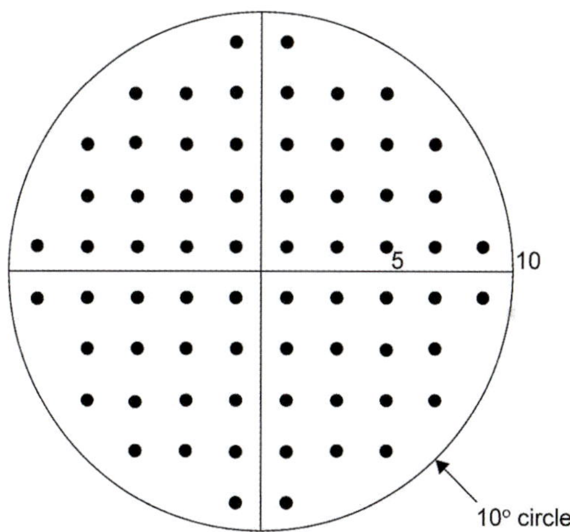

Fig. 3: Displays the points tested in the 10-2 program on Humphrey visual field (HVF).

Various threshold testing strategies got introduced from time to time to yield better results. Perimetry being a subjective test, a lot depends on the patient's performance. The testing threshold strategies are as follows:

- Full Threshold strategy (1983)
- FAST PAC (1991)
- SITA Standard (1997)
- SITA Fast (1997)

The full threshold is a very long test as it involves a 4-2 bracketing strategy. The FAST PAC reduces the time by 40% as compared to the Full Threshold.

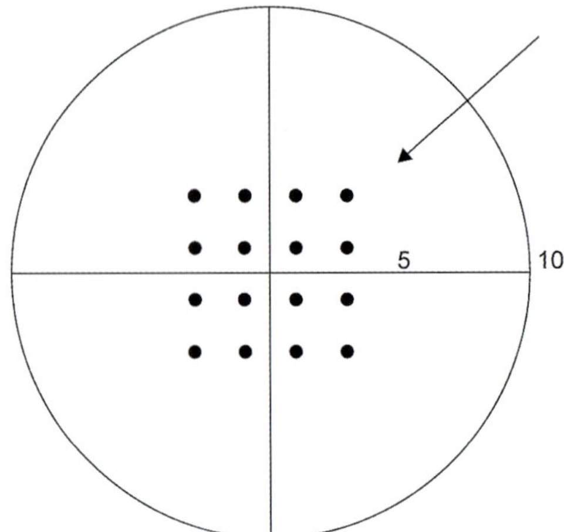

Fig. 4: Displays points tested on the macular program on Humphrey visual field (HVF).

Here the test uses a 3 dB change instead of 4 dB and crosses the threshold only once.

The SITA Standard and the SITA FAST calculate expected thresholds and are thus able to begin testing close to the actual threshold. They use the patient's normative data, which is constantly updated. Sita standard takes half the time of standard full threshold. SITA FAST takes half the time of FAST PAC. The Pace of the test is dependent on patient's response time.

Newly added 24-2C Sita Faster tests have 10 additional central points from the 10-2 in addition to the 54 points tested in 24-2, to ensure it does not miss any central defect. These points are placed in both the hemifields equally. The 24-2C Sita Faster is significantly faster than both 24-2 and 10-2 tests, reducing the testing time by 46 and 52%, respectively. It has proven to be highly effective in detecting mild stage glaucoma with central visual field.

Normally perimetry printouts have two kinds of data, one with STATPAC analysis and the other without any STATPAC analysis.

- Raw DATA without STATPAC analysis
- Macular Program
- Nasal Step Printout
- Stimulus V tests
- Raw DATA with STATPAC analysis
- Single Field Analysis Printout
- Change Analysis Printout
- Glaucoma Change Probability Analysis
- Glaucoma Progression Analysis (GPA)

How does one do an analysis of a single field printout?

This is a typical printout. To get maximum out of the data provided in this printout, it is best to divide the printout into eight zones as shown in **Figure 5**.

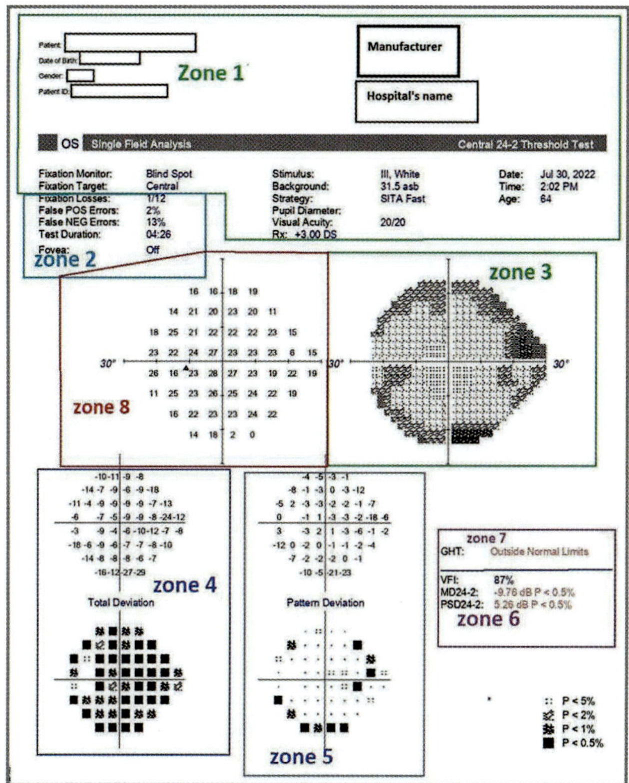

Fig. 5: A normal printout of a 30-2 Humphrey visual field (HVF) and how to divide it into eight zones to read an individual printout.

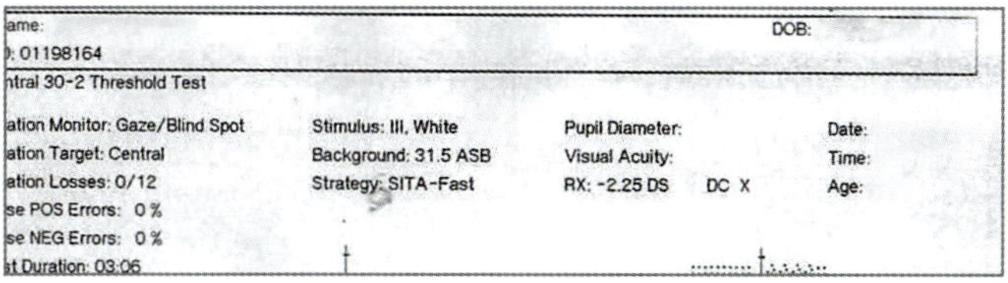

ame: DOB:
): 01198164
ntral 30-2 Threshold Test

ation Monitor: Gaze/Blind Spot | Stimulus: III, White | Pupil Diameter: | Date:
ation Target: Central | Background: 31.5 ASB | Visual Acuity: | Time:
ation Losses: 0/12 | Strategy: SITA-Fast | RX: -2.25 DS DC X | Age:
se POS Errors: 0 %
se NEG Errors: 0 %
st Duration: 03:06

Fig. 6: Zone 1: Patient test details.

If you follow this order, you will have looked at everything you need to, in the correct perspective and cannot make a mistake in interpretation.

Let us see how we start. Look at zone 1. This zone normally gives you the patient test details. It tells you the test done, the strategy used, the stimulus size, the eye that is tested, the visual acuity, the age of the patient, and the date the test was performed. It also gives you the pupillary diameter **(Fig. 6)**.

Move on to zone 2, which shows the reliability factors **(Box 1)**.

BOX 1: Reliability factors.

- Fixation monitor: Gaze/blind spot
- *Fixation target:* Central
- *Fixation losses:* 1/16
- *False POS errors:* 6%
- *False NEG errors:* 1%
- *Test duration:* 05:01
- *Fovea:* 36 dB

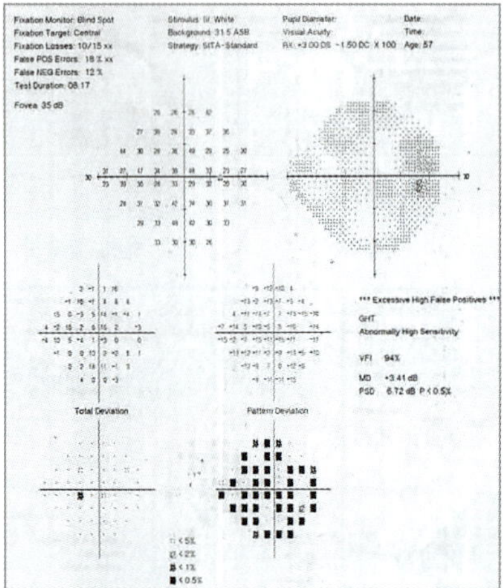

Fig. 7: False positives.

It shows the fixation losses, to see how steady the patient's fixation has been. It also gives the false-negative and false-positive responses. A false-negative response is one, where the patient is inattentive, tired, and does not press the button, even if he see the stimulus. The false-positive responses are normally seen in trigger happy patients, who press the button even without seeing a stimulus. Up to 20% of these responses are alright to do an interpretation, anything beyond, makes the printout unreliable. In the patients who show too many false negatives, in the gray scale you see what typically shows a clover leaf pattern, where the patient is alert in the beginning and then loses interest. In the printout where there are too many false positives, you see white scotoma, so the threshold sensitivity can be as high as 40 dB. Fixation losses have to be monitored, so that we know the visual field has been done with the patient keeping his gaze steady on the fixation point. Fixation monitoring is done using the Heijl–Krakau method, where 5% of the stimuli are presented on the blind spot. The patient's response to this stimulus is due to shift of fixation. It also indicates shift of gaze. The fixation losses >20% are considered to be unreliable **(Figs. 7 and 8)**.

Now we move on to the zone 3, which presents the numerical raw data in a graphical form. The retinal sensitivity values from 0 to 50 dB are divided into 10 groups. Each step of the pattern corresponds to a change of 5 dB intensity, except the first column represented by 41–50 dB **(Fig. 9)**.

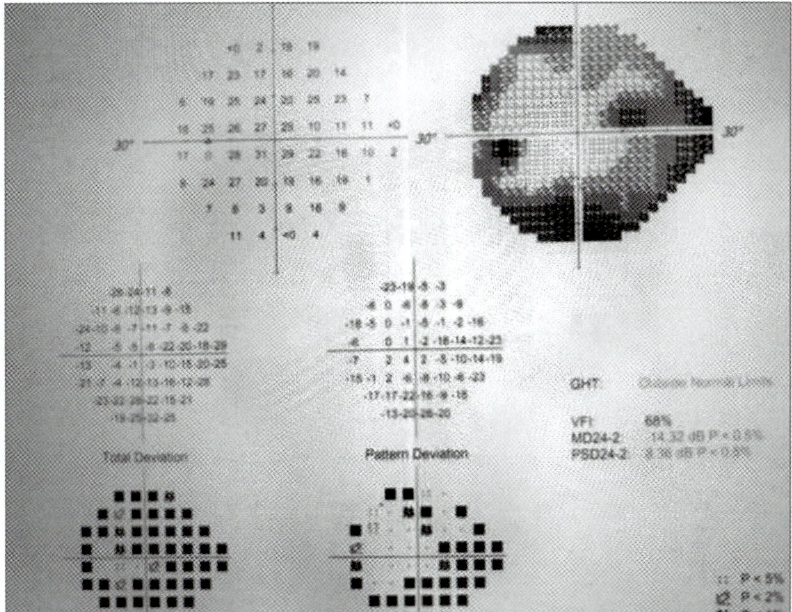

Fig. 8: False negatives.

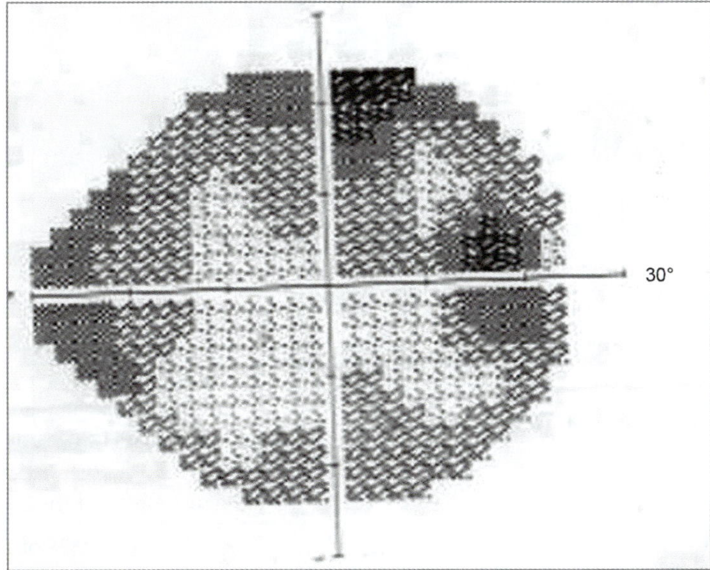

Fig. 9: Gray scale/zone 3.

Zone 4 raw data is compared with the mean normal retinal sensitivity of those points of the age-matched normals. The STATPAC calculates the difference between them at each point and plots them as total deviation numerical plot **(Fig. 10)**.

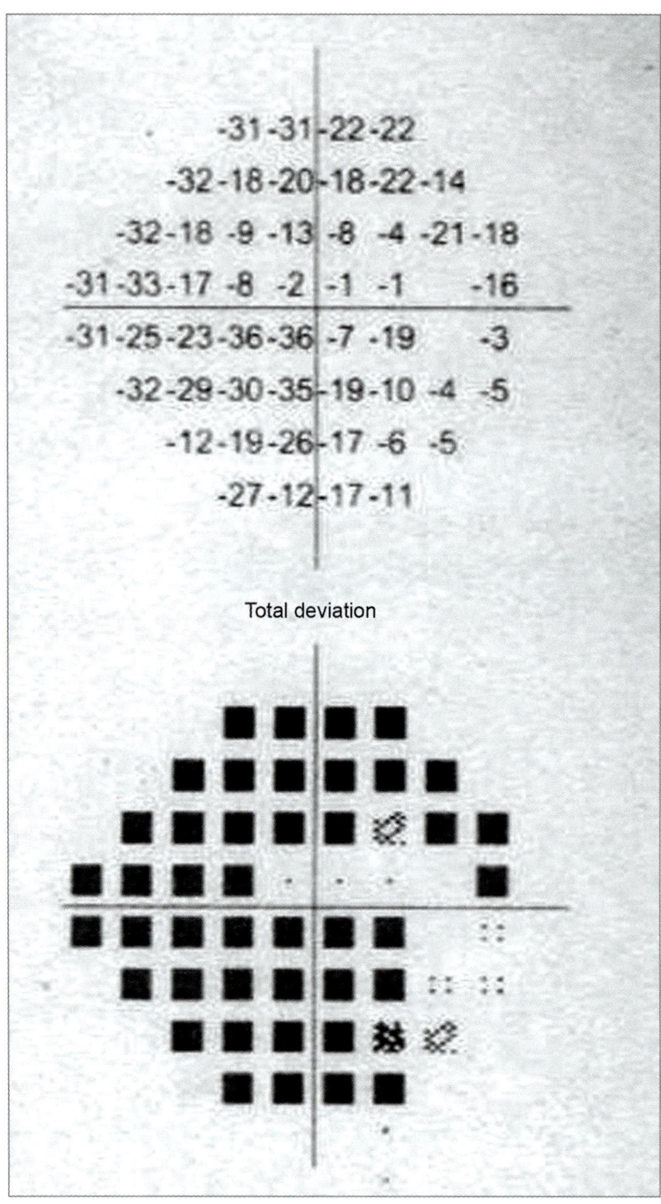

Fig. 10: Zone 4/total deviation plot.

Notes:
- P <5% indicates the retinal sensitivity of that point is seen in <5% of normal population.
- P <2% indicates the retinal sensitivity of that point is seen in <2% of normal population.
- P <1% indicates the retinal sensitivity of that point is seen in <1% of normal population.
- P <0.5% indicates the retinal sensitivity of that point is seen in <0.5% of normal population.

Moving on to the next zone, that is zone 5, that is the pattern deviation plot. It also shows the pattern deviation probability plot.

The main function of pattern deviation plot is to expose localized defects that may be masked by either a generalized depression or an elevation of the hill of vision **(Figs. 11 to 15)**.

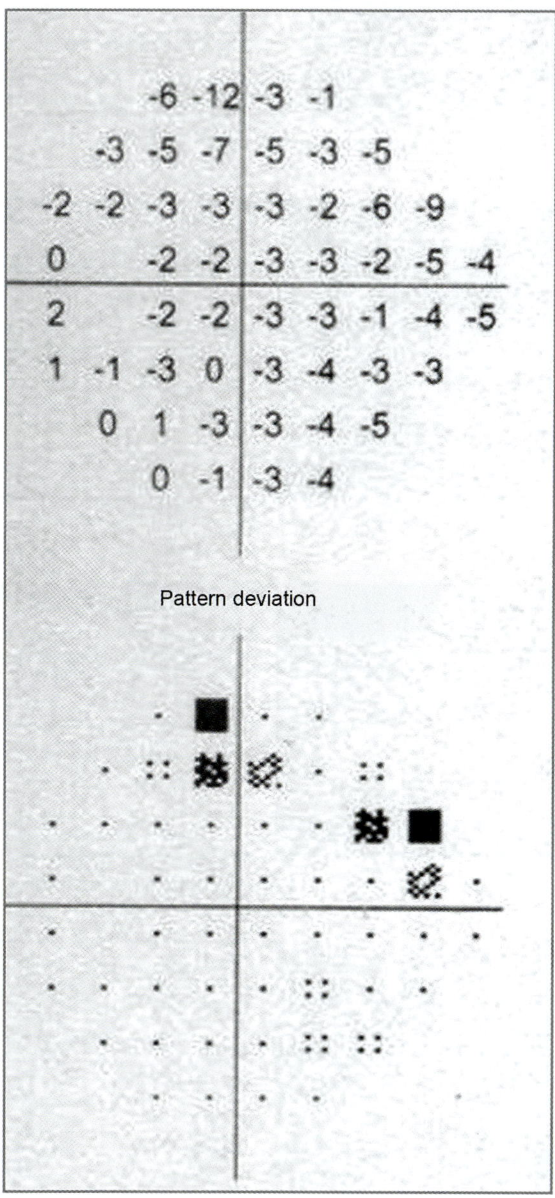

Fig. 11: Zone 5/pattern standard deviation plot, also includes the probability plot.

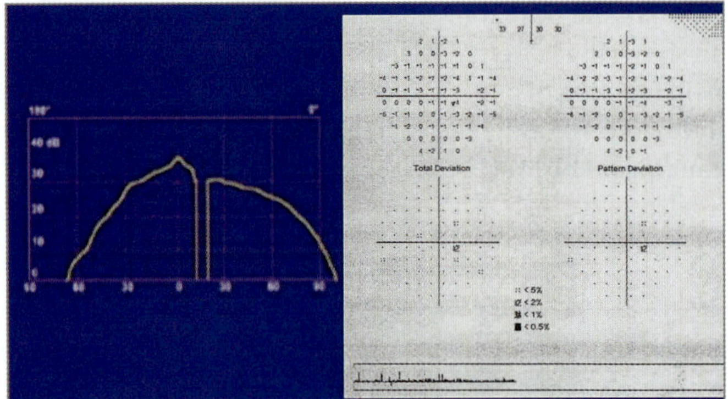

Fig. 12: Normal hill of vision.

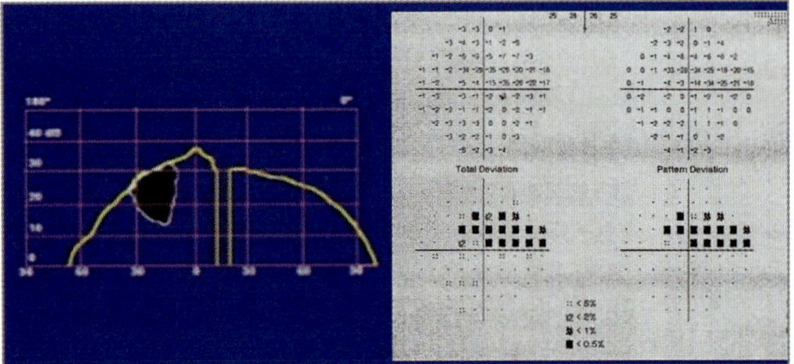

Fig. 13: Normal hill of vision with a localized scotoma.

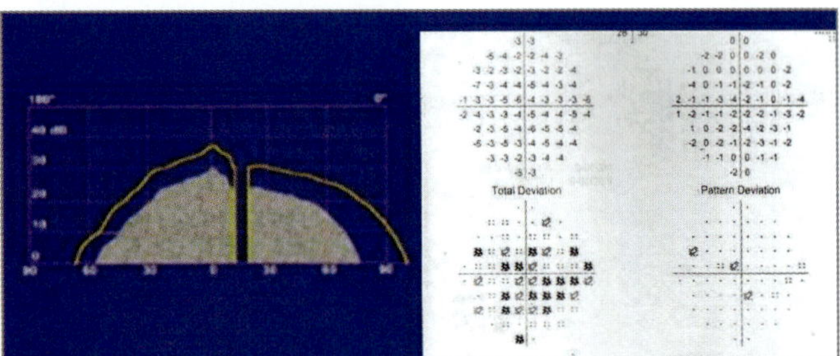

Fig. 14: Hill of vision with a generalized depression.

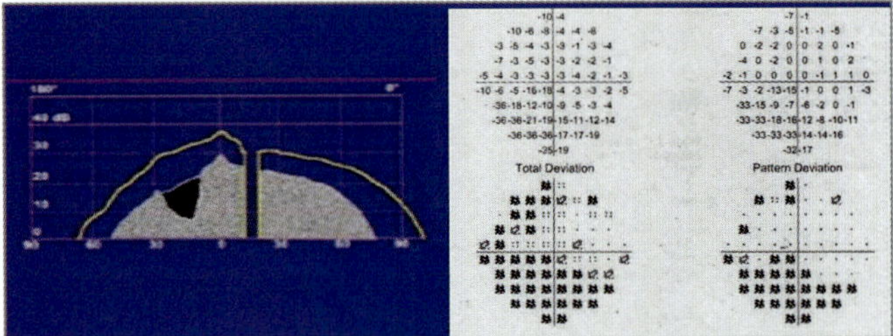

Fig. 15: Generalized depression with a localized scotoma.

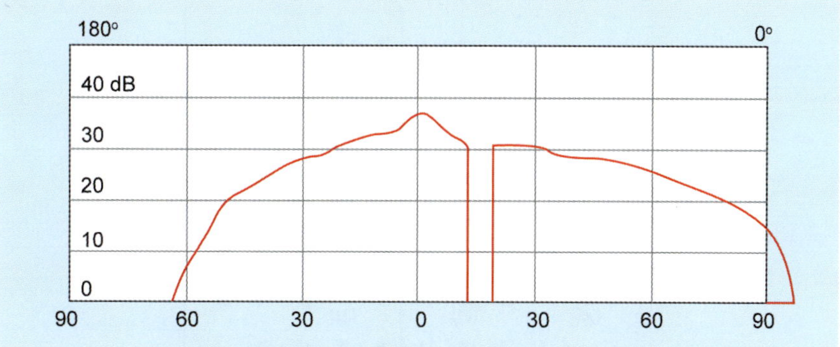

Fig. 16: Two dimensional view of the field of vision.

MD	–23.82 dB P < 0.5%
PSD	11.74 dB P < 0.5%
SF	3.13 dB P < 2%
CPSD	11.25 dB P < 0.5%

Fig. 17: Global indices.

Zone 6, the next zone, shows us the global indices. These are statistical calculations helping us interpret. They show us the following parameters **(Figs. 16 and 17)**:

- Mean deviation (MD)
- Pattern standard deviation (PSD)
- Short-term fluctuation (SF)
- Corrected pattern standard deviation (CPSD)
    - *MD:* It expresses the change in the height of hill of vision
    - *PSD:* It expresses the change in smoothness of the contour of the hill of vision.
    - *SFs:* It is an index of intratest variation. At 10 preselected points, the retinal sensitivity will be calculated twice. The result of the first and second value is compared; so high SF sometimes indicates pathology and sometimes index of unreliability **(Fig. 18)**.
    - It is also used to correct PSD to produce CPSD.
    - *CPSD or corrected pattern standard deviation:* It is calculated as an adjustment to the PSD after adjusting for short-term fluctuations. The intratesting variability (SF) is removed from PSD to produce CPSD.

Zone 7 shows a very important parameter called the *Glaucoma Hemifield Test (GHT)*

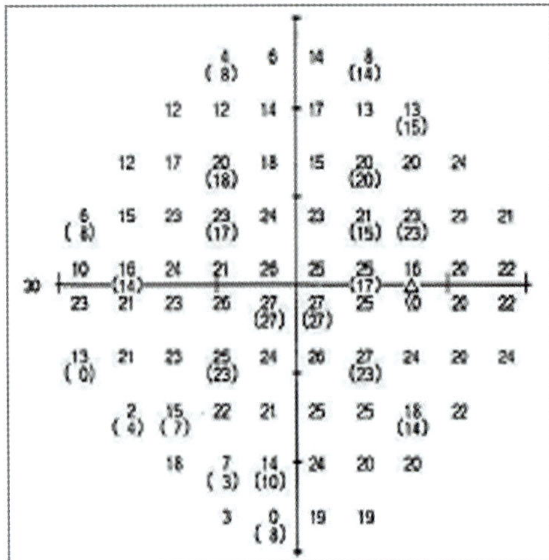

Fig. 18: How short-term fluctuations are tested.

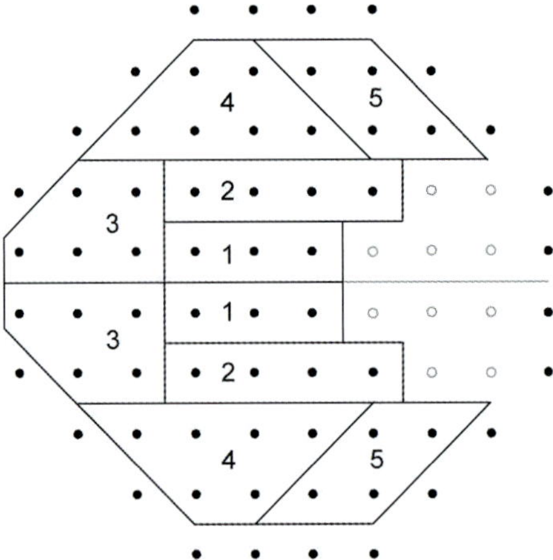

Fig. 19: Glaucoma hemifield test showing five sets of numbers above the horizontal meridian are compared to mirror images below the horizontal meridian.

Here, five set of points above the horizontal meridian are compared to mirror image below the horizontal meridian as shown in **Figure 19** and the results are shown in print as shown below:

- *Outside normal limits:*
  - All cluster pairs differ @ $p < 1\%$ OR
  - One cluster pair differs @ $p < 0.5\%$
- *Borderline:* Hemifields differ @ $p < 3\%$
- *General reduction of sensitivity:* Overall field depressed @ $p < 0.5\%$
- *Abnormal high sensitivity:* Overall field elevated (best 15% points) @ $p < 0.5\%$
- Within normal limits

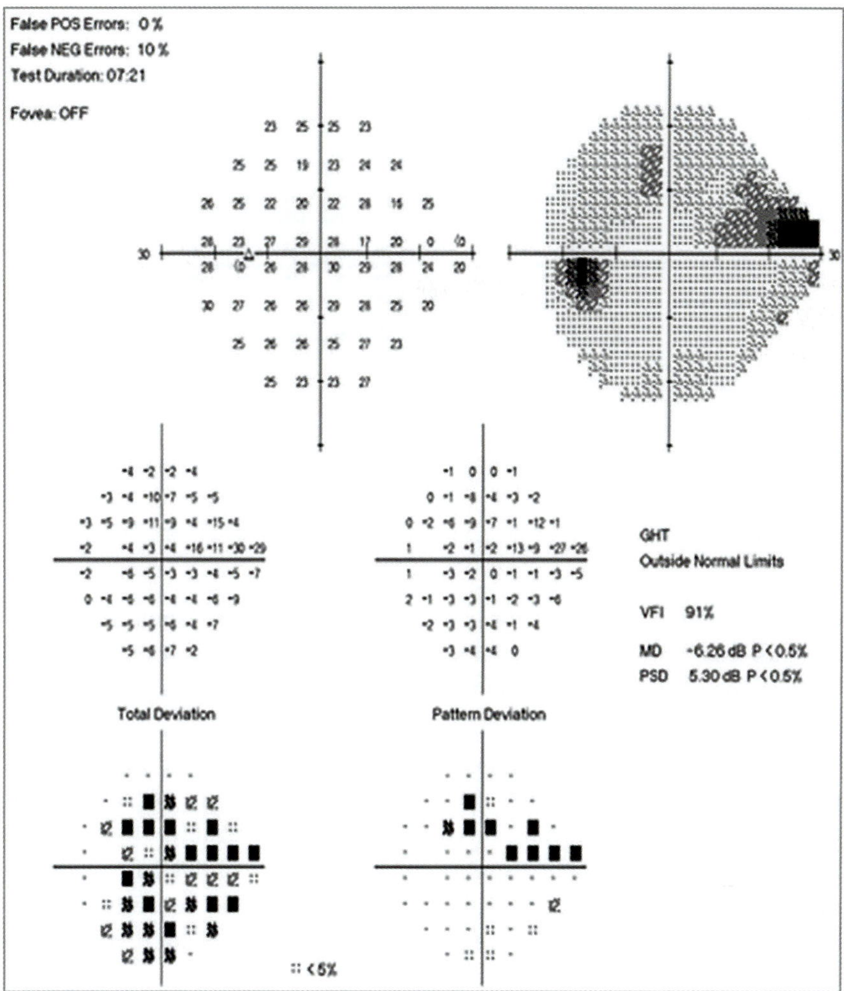

Fig. 20: Visual field index (VFI), seen in % of normal age-corrected sensitivity.

Visual field index (VFI) is a single figure and a relatively new parameter included in the global indices. It is a single number that summarizes each patient's visual field status as a percentage of normal age-corrected sensitivity. It reflects the rate of ganglion cell loss and is derived from PD and is center weighted **(Fig. 20)**.

The next and the last zone for interpretation is the Raw Data. The Raw Data is the exact retinal sensitivity in dB units of the selected points calculated by field analyzer **(Fig. 21)**.

Even though the interpretation looks very simple following this method, there still exist some sources of error which include *miosis*, which decreases the sensitivity in the peripheral field of vision, and may increase the variability

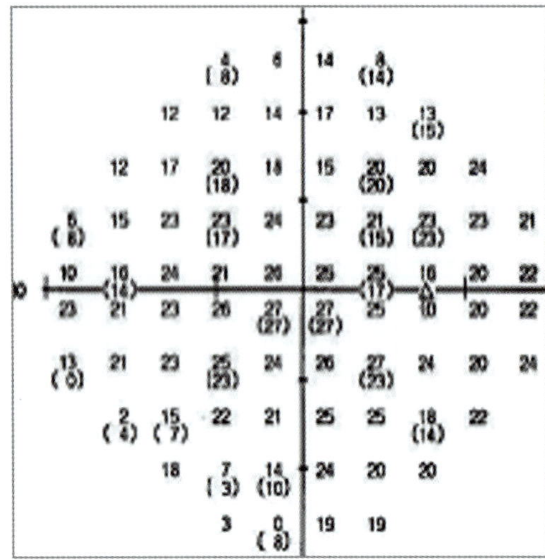

Fig. 21: Raw Data, the actual retinal sensitivity at the points tested in dB.

in central field of vision. *Uncorrected refractive error*: Threshold sensitivity appears less. Spectacles can cause rim scotomas. *Ptosis*: It can result in suppression of inferior visual field. An *unsteady patient* or an *anxious patient* can make subjective errors and hence the test needs to be patiently explained to this patient. The perimetrist needs to be very patient and gets the best performance from the patient. Due to this reason, it is not uncommon for the patients to have a learning curve in doing the test reliably. There may be inconsistent and unreliable responses on first test. The initial field may show overall reduced sensitivity (negative MD). Interpretation becomes difficult and progression may not be judged until the patient has not learnt to produce stable baseline effect.

How do you diagnose that a particular defect is glaucomatous?

There are Anderson's criteria to diagnose glaucoma **(Fig. 22)***:*

In the *pattern deviation plot*, look for:

- 3 contiguous non-edge points with $p < 5\%$
- 1 point with $p < 1\%$.
- The cluster in must be in an arcuate area.
- *CPSD:* $p < 5\%$ on two consecutive fields
- *GHT:* Outside normal limits on at least two fields

PROGRESSION ON PERIMETRY

It is a long topic, which needs a chapter on its own, but we will just touch upon the most salient features that one needs to know. *What is progression?* Obviously, it is a change in state from an earlier stage to the next one. We are all

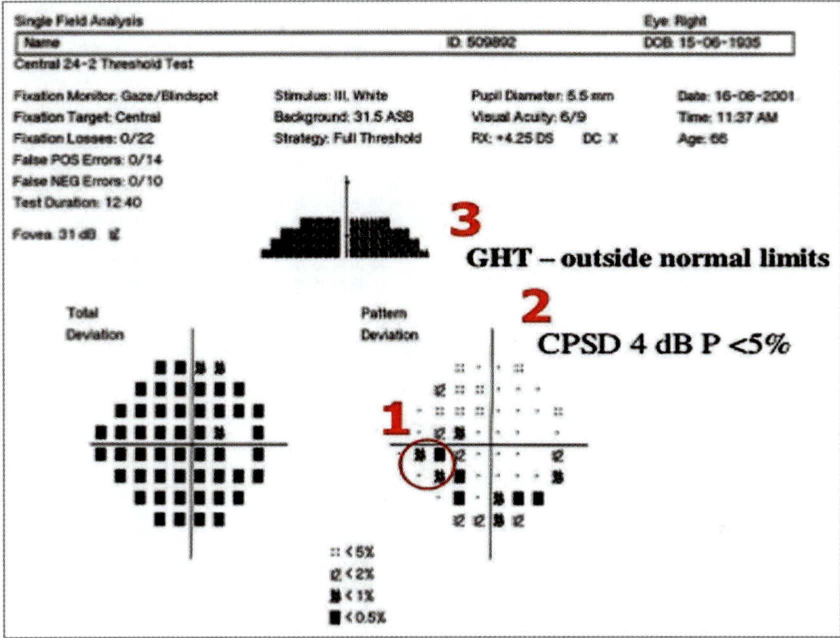

Fig. 22: Anderson's criteria showing how to identify a defect is due to glaucoma.

aware of the "continuum of glaucoma". So when you move on from one stage of the continuum to the next, it is progression. To determine progression, you must have stable, baseline fields, hence two baseline fields are a must. The existing defect can increase in size, or in depth or a new defect can come up. All of these scenarios describe progression, however, there are many factors that can interfere with our ability to detect progression. There may be a long-term fluctuation. The patient may not be able to do a reliable field once in a way. A new artifact can crop up on 1 day. All of these are hindrances in detecting progression.

A rough estimate of looking at progression can be to compare successive fields with one another, known as the overview printouts. However, statistical analysis is not provided in this way. It is almost a mere eyeballing of the gray scales, as shown in **Figure 23**.

Then came the Change Analysis Printout, where a display up to 16 fields at a time were studied. Three components: (1) a box plot with its relation to the dB scale, (2) the summary of the global indices, and (3) the linear regression analysis of MD. Indices are plotted overtime to indicate the changes in the patient's visual field **(Fig. 24)**.

The glaucoma change probability analysis is designed to facilitate interpretation of central 30-2 and central 24-2 threshold follow-up tests in patients with suspect or manifest glaucoma **(Fig. 25)**.

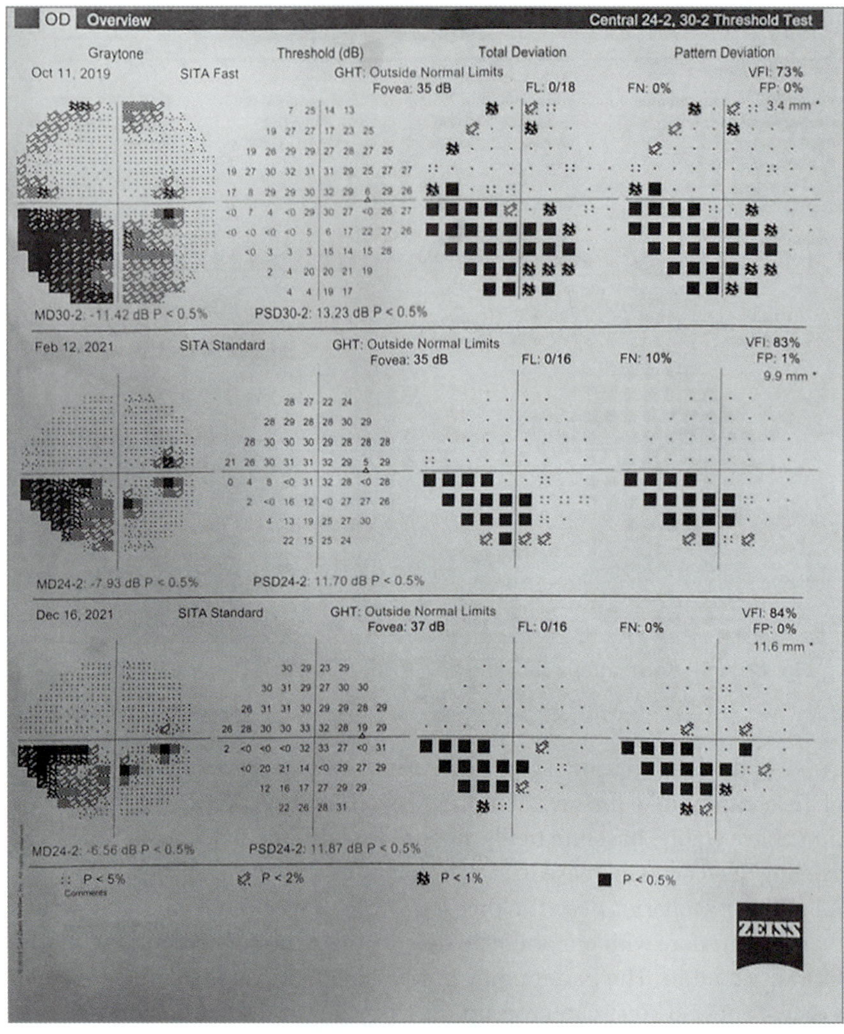

Fig. 23: Overview printout to look for progression with consecutive fields seen together, to get an overall impression of change.

Follow three steps in this interpretation:

- *Step 1:* Establishing the baseline data (total deviation numerical plot)
- *Step 2:* Establishing the decibel deviation plot
- *Step 3:* Establishing the change probability plot (compares rate of change in patient's visual field with stable glaucoma patient)

There are four symbols which help you interpret the change:

1. *Solid dots:* No significant change in sensitivity as compared to baseline
2. *Half-filled triangles:* Progression at 95% significance level

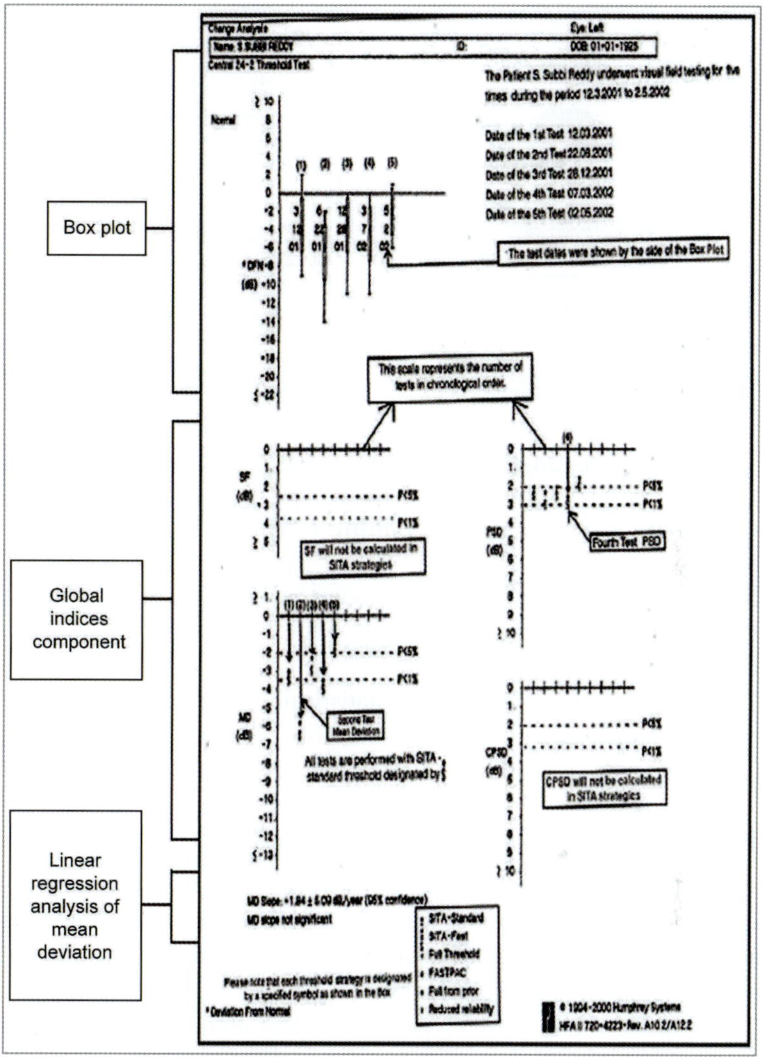

Box plot

Global indices component

Linear regression analysis of mean deviation

Change Analysis Eye: Left

Central 24-2 Threshold Test

The Patient S. Subbi Reddy underwent visual field testing for five times during the period 12.3.2001 to 2.5.2002

Date of the 1st Test 12.03.2001
Date of the 2nd Test 22.08.2001
Date of the 3rd Test 28.12.2001
Date of the 4th Test 07.03.2002
Date of the 5th Test 02.05.2002

The test dates were shown by the side of the Box Plot

This scale represents the number of tests in chronological order.

SF will not be calculated in SITA strategies

Fourth Test PSD

Second Test Mean Deviation

All tests are performed with SITA-standard threshold designated by $

CPSD will not be calculated in SITA strategies

MD Slope: +1.84 ± 5.00 dB/year (95% confidence)
MD slope not significant

Please note that each threshold strategy is designated by a specified symbol as shown in the box

* Deviation From Normal

SITA-Standard
SITA-Fast
Full Threshold
FASTPAC
Full from prior
Reduced reliability

© 1994-2000 Humphrey Systems

Fig. 24: Change Analysis printout.

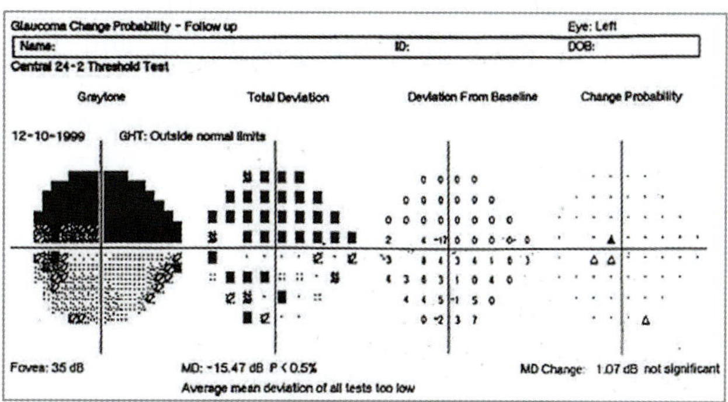

Fig. 25: Glaucoma change probability analysis.

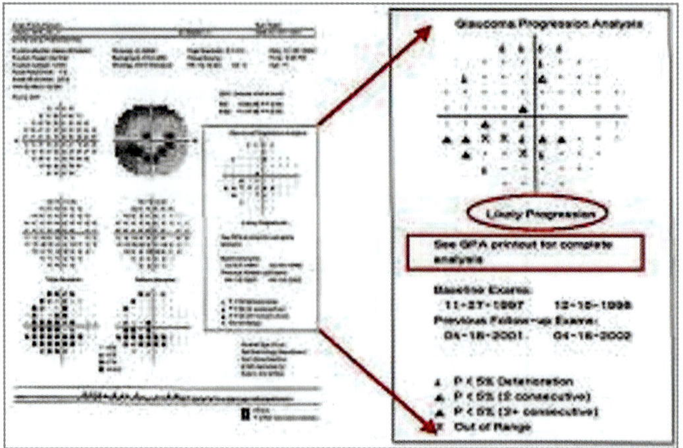

Fig. 26: Glaucoma Progression Analysis (GPA).

3. *Open triangles:* Progression point repeated in two consecutive examinations
4. *Black solid triangles:* Progression point repeated in three consecutive examinations
5. *Cross:* Out of range

The *GPA* is the newer version of a statistically aided program. In GPA, the comparisons are made between the baseline pattern deviation numerical plot and the pattern deviation numerical plot of the follow-up test **(Fig. 26)**.

IN THE EVENT-BASED PROGRESSION

Any change has occurred and whether it is statistically significant. The differences in visual field sensitivities of the current tests are compared to those of previously established baseline examinations and the prints give you possible progression, likely progression **(Fig. 27)**.

Trend-based analysis gives you the rate of change and its statistical significance. It is based on linear regression of the VFI over time **(Fig. 28)**.

The criteria for change are based on the following factors:

- *Minimum of three tests required:* Two baseline and one follow-up examination
- Each follow-up compared to averaged thresholds of two baseline examinations
- Additional follow-up compared both to baseline and to two most recent follow-ups
- Progressing point repeated in two consecutive examinations: possible progression
- Progressing point repeated in three consecutive examinations: likely progression

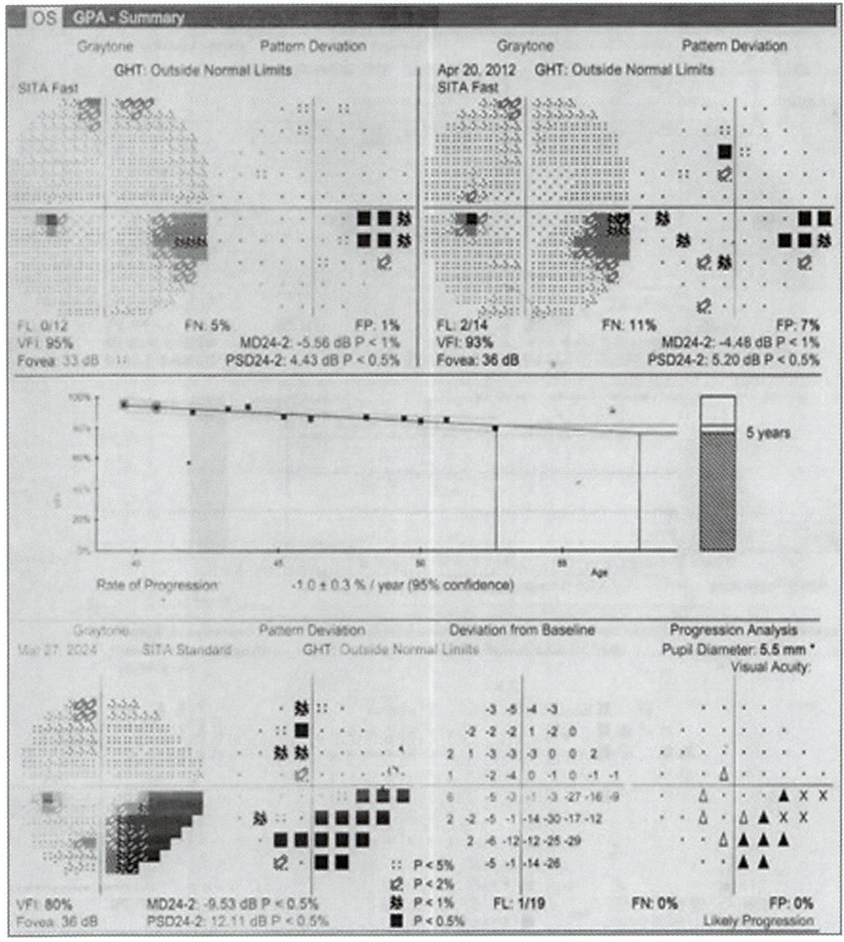

Fig. 27: Event-based progression.

GPA alert: Three in one examination denotes "Possible Progression" and two indicates "Likely Progression" **(Figs. 29 and 30)**.

Going to the first automated perimeter, it was Fankhauser, Spahr, and Jenni in 1974 who introduced the Octopus 201. It has been upgraded many times since then, but the honor of introducing this form of perimetry certainly belongs to the *Octopus*.

There is a difference in the way fixation is monitored between the two major perimeters too.

In the OCTOPUS perimeter, the target is at the center of the pupil, which is projected in the display. The fixation monitor is automatically controlled and, hence, it stops projecting when the patient loses fixation and promptly resumes when the fixation is back on target. Here, therefore there is a 100% eye fixation control **(Tables 2 and 3)**.

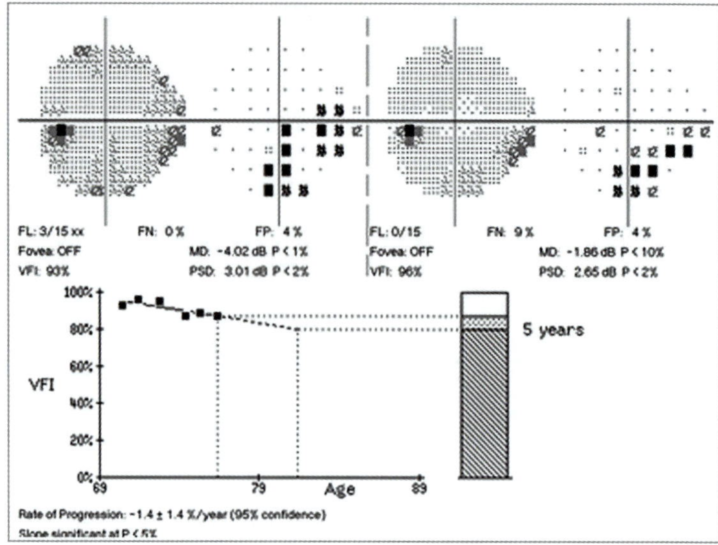

Fig. 28: Trend-based analysis of progression.

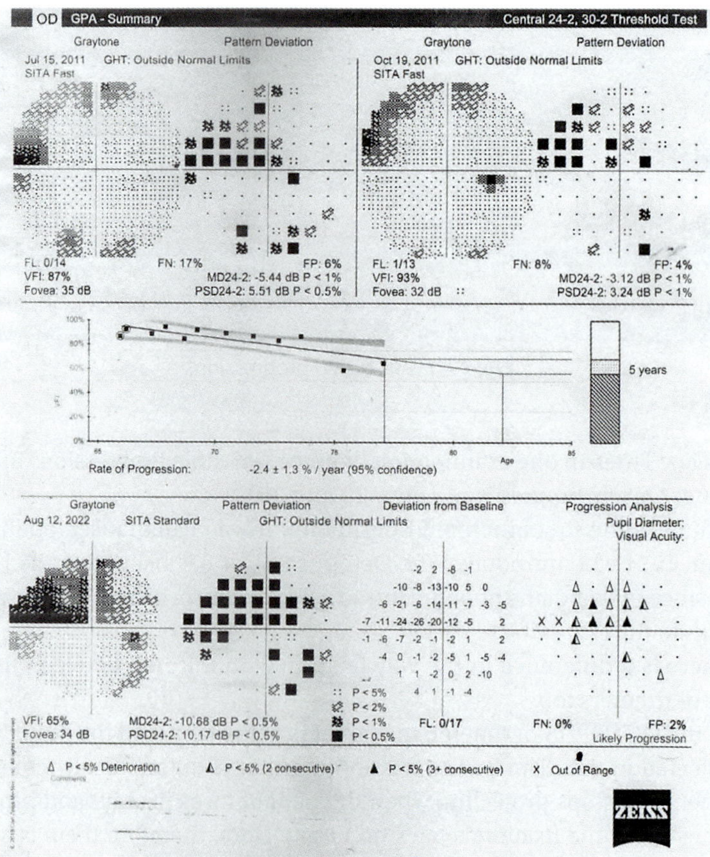

Fig. 29: Glaucoma Progression Analysis (GPA) alert.

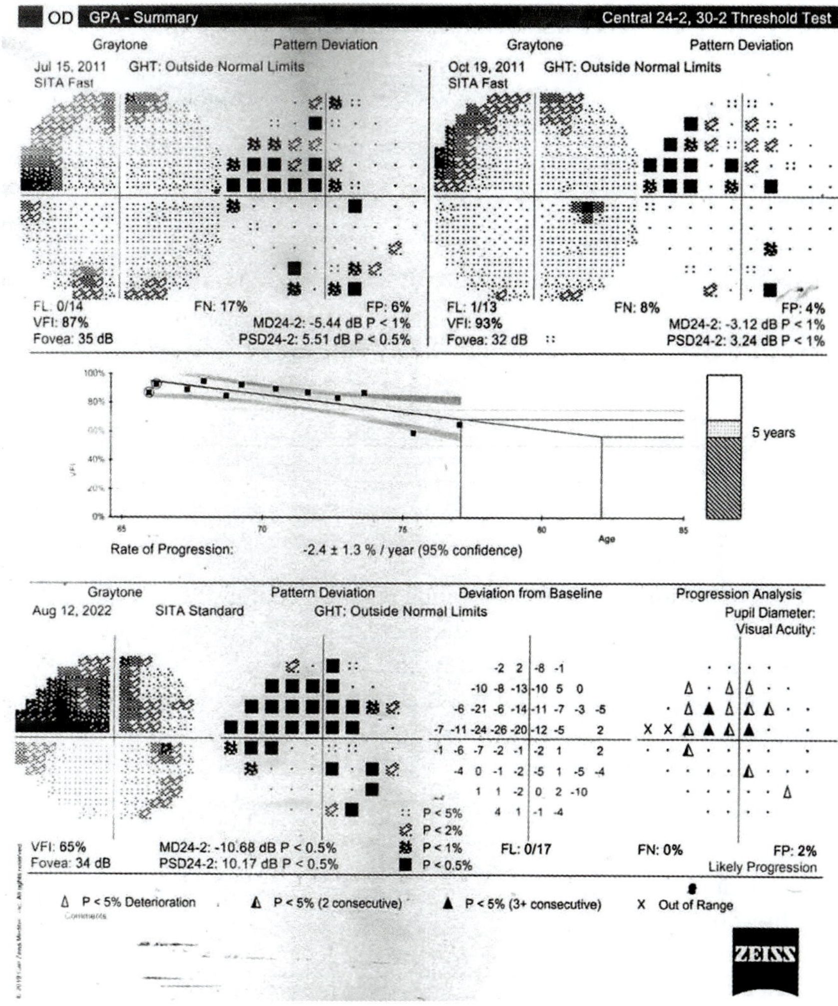

Fig. 30: Glaucoma Progression Analysis (GPA) summary.

TABLE 2: The difference in the illumination between Octopus and Humphrey.

Apostilbs and decibels on the Humphrey and Octopus perimeters		
Apostilbs	***Humphrey decibels***	***Octopus decibels***
0.1	50	40
1	40	30
10	30	20
100	20	10
1,000	10	0
10,000	0	

TABLE 3: The difference between the stimulus in the Humphrey and Octopus perimeter.

Variable	*Humphrey field analyzer*	*Octopus perimeter*
Stimulus size	III and V	• III and V in Octopus 1-2-3 • I to V in Octopus 101
Stimulus	White or red	White
Minimum stimulus intensity	0.1 asb	0.1 asb
Maximum stimulus intensity	10,000 asb	6,000 asb
Stimulus duration	200 milliseconds	100 milliseconds

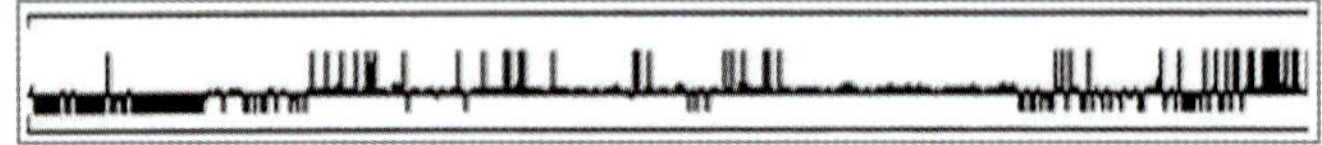

Fig. 31: Gaze tracker tracing.

In the Humphrey as against that there is a gaze tracker. Every movement of the eye fixation off the target, which is at the center of the pupil, shows up as an upward spike on the tracing. Here, again the fixation monitor loses fixation, when the eye moves away and resumes fixation when fixation resumes. When the patient blinks, it is recorded as a downward spike on the tracing. Fixation losses are measured by the Heijl-Krakau method and displayed in the printout **(Fig. 31)**.

Like the Humphrey, the Octopus too has its own testing strategies, which are as follows:

- Screening strategies
- Threshold strategies
- Full threshold strategy
- Fast threshold strategy
- Dynamic test strategy
- Tendency-oriented perimetry (TOP)
- Staging and phasing technology

Just like the Humphrey to reduce the testing time, the OCTOPUS strategy uses the dynamic strategy, which reduces the test time by 30–40%. It does this when the depth of defect is deep, the step sizes increases from increment steps of 2–10 dB to achieve final calculated value from the last two tested values **(Figs. 32A and B)**.

In the TOP or the tendency-oriented perimetry, each test location is assessed only once and the subject's response at that location is used to assess not only sensitivity at that point but also to modify the current sensitivity estimate of neighboring locations reduces test time to 2.5–3 minutes **(Fig. 33)**.

In staging, priority is given to the locations of importance depending on the diagnosis.

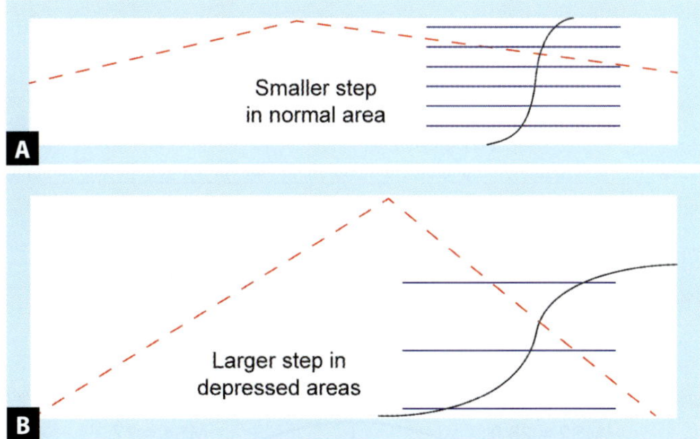

Figs. 32A and B: (A) Routine testing strategy in the Octopus; (B) Dynamic testing strategy in Octopus to reduce testing time.

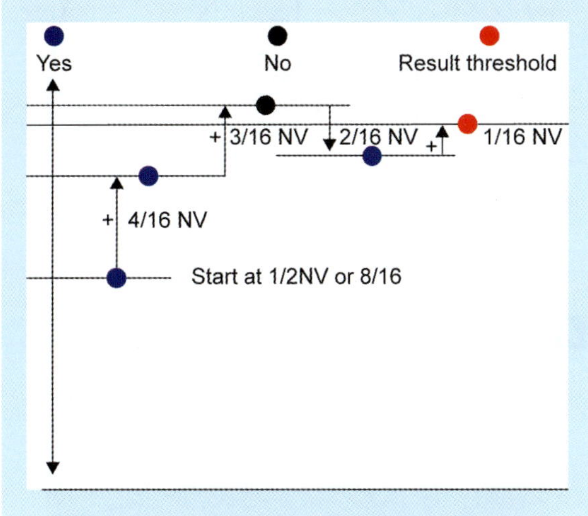

Fig. 33: Tendency-oriented perimetry (TOP).

Allows examination of more relevant areas when the patient is fresh. In phasing, the following can be done **(Fig. 34)**:

- Test may be saved, printed, or stopped
- *Retested:* Short-term fluctuation
- Quantify relative defects
- Extend the field area by skipping test in center and continuing in periphery

Let us see the G1/2 program on the Octopus. Both are identical in central 30°. 59 test points are tested. In the G2 program, an additional 15 test points in 30–60° test locations respect the topography of nerve fiber layer. Foveal and paracentral areas have resolution: 2.8° **(Figs. 35A and B)**.

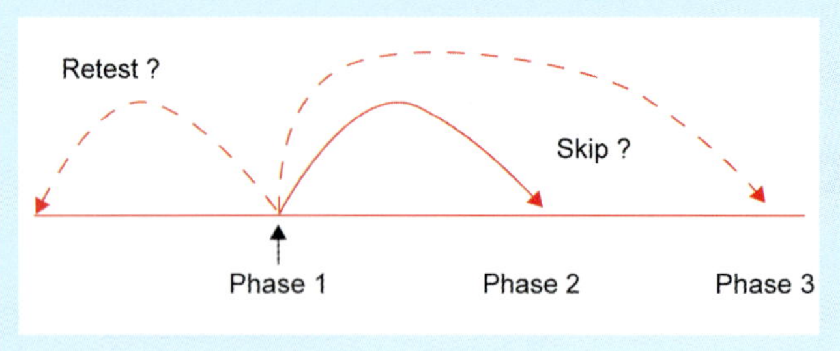

Fig. 34: Phasing.

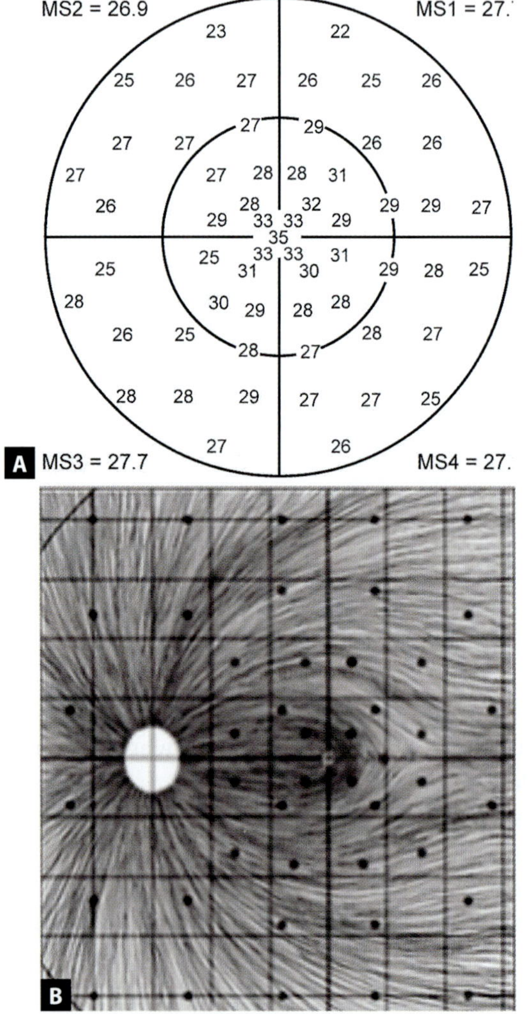

Figs. 35A and B: G1 Program on the Octopus points are tested along the maculopapillary bundle.

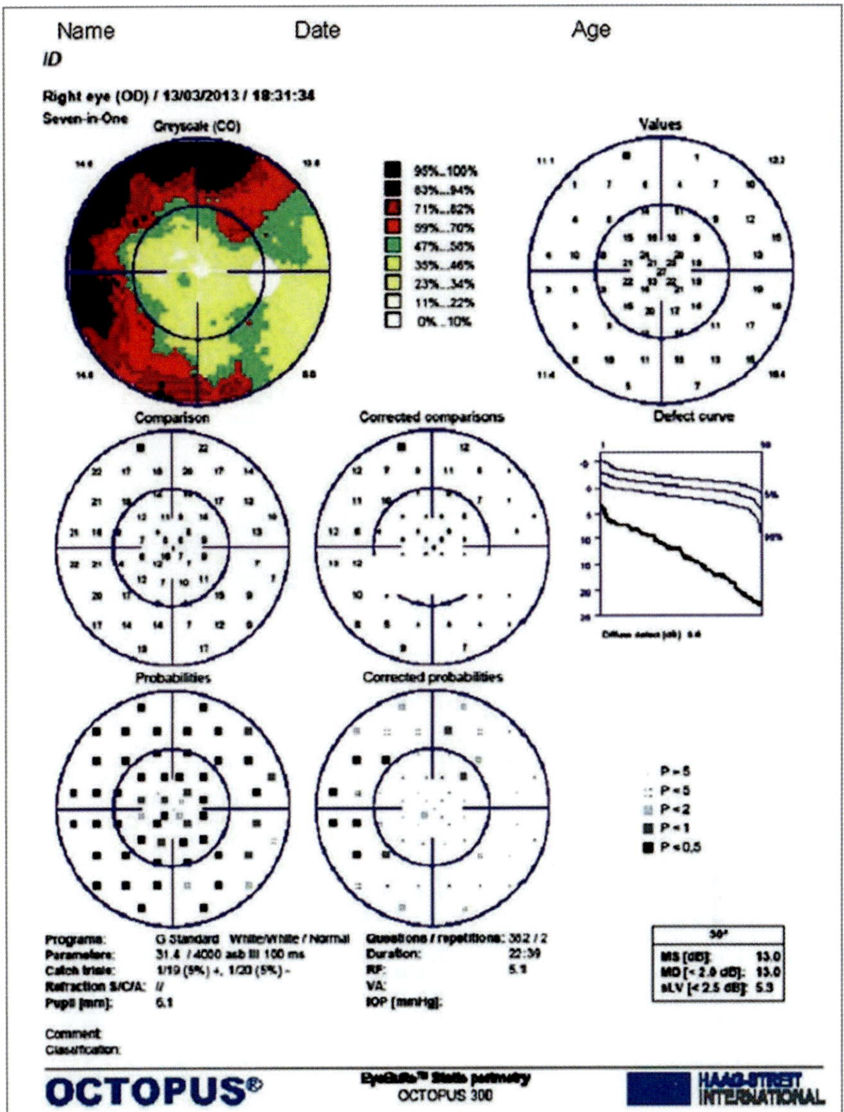

Fig. 36: Octopus printout.

Both the printouts look pretty similar only with changes in nomenclature **(Figs. 36 and 37)**.

The total deviation in the Humphrey is called comparisons in the Octopus printout, the pattern standard deviation in the Humphrey is called corrected comparisons. There is no GHT in the Octopus, but is replaced with a *Bebie curve*. It is a cumulative defect curve that allows ranking of visual field defects (it looks only at the defects, not the field). It is used to rank visual field defects and distinguish between localized and diffuse damage. It is a clinical data

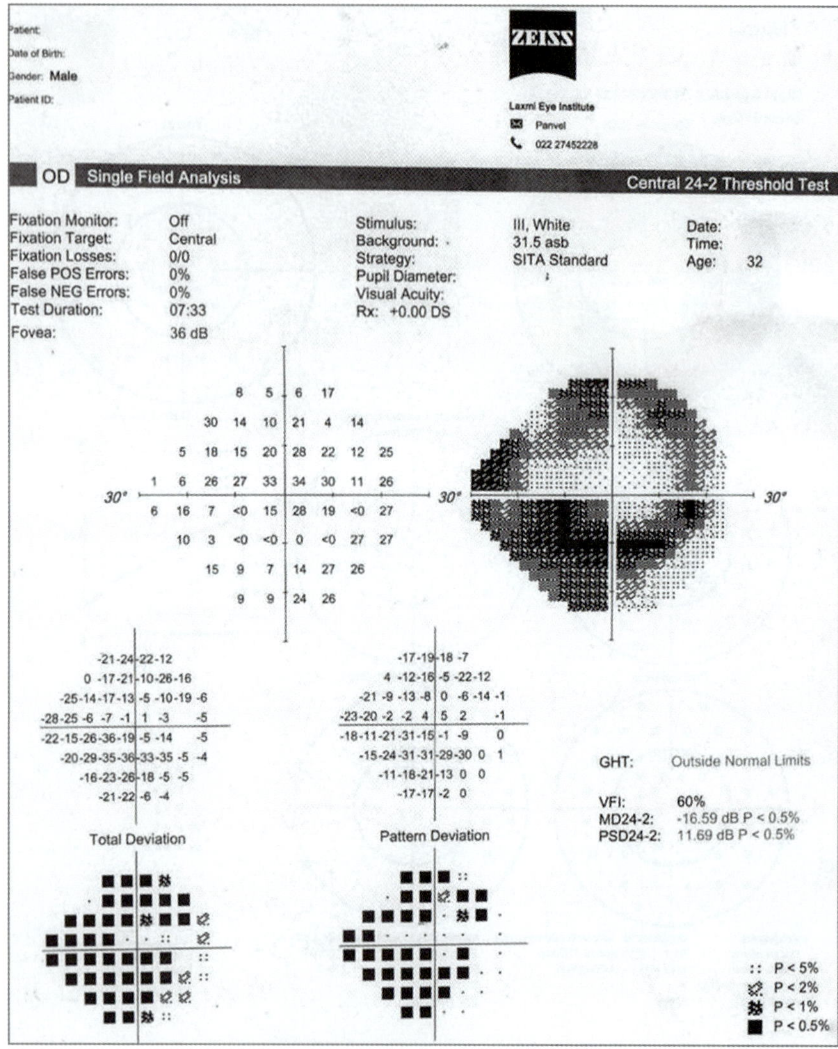

Fig. 37: Humphrey printout.

representation procedure that can be used to evaluate visual fields for ocular and neurologic disorders. The Bebie curve can be used to classify the severity of glaucoma, monitor disease progression, and adjust therapy. It can also be used to describe visual field conditions in a simple format. This curve can help to recognize diffuse damage in the visual field, which can be difficult to quantify in the presence of scotomas **(Fig. 38)**.

Let us compare the *global indices* of the two machines, the *mean deviation* in the *Humphrey* is represented by the *mean defect (MD)* in the *Octopus*. MD (Octopus) stands for arithmetic mean of the difference between the values measured in the examination and that of the age-matched normals.

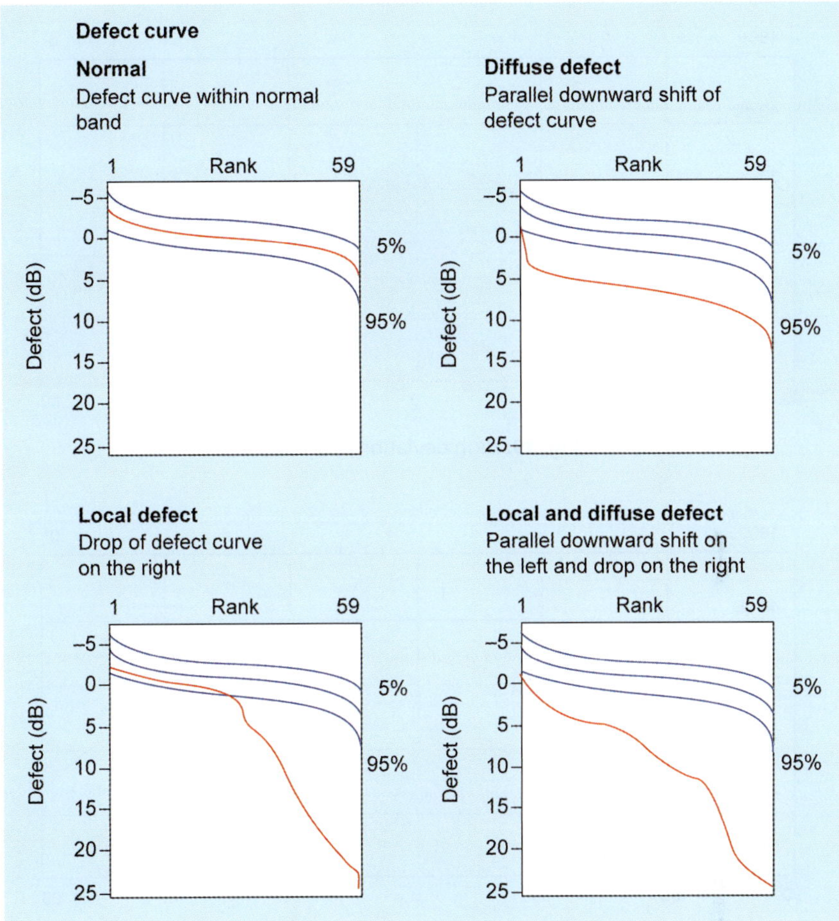

Fig. 38: Bebie curve showing normal, diffuse defect, local defect, and a local defect with a diffuse defect.

A positive value indicates depression. The *mean sensitivity* in the *Octopus* is the arithmetic mean of the threshold determined at all of the points in that field. The *loss variance* in the *Octopus* stands for the *pattern standard deviation* in the Humphrey. It basically expresses the change in smoothness of the contour of the hill of vision. In a uniformly distributed field, the local visual (LV)/PSD is small. In localized defects, the LV/PSD tends to be high **(Figs. 39 and 40)**.

Progression in the Octopus visual field is analyzed by two ways:

1. Cluster analysis
2. Polar trends

Cluster analysis: Typical glaucomatous defects always occur in a cluster of adjacent defective visual field locations that correspond to the path followed

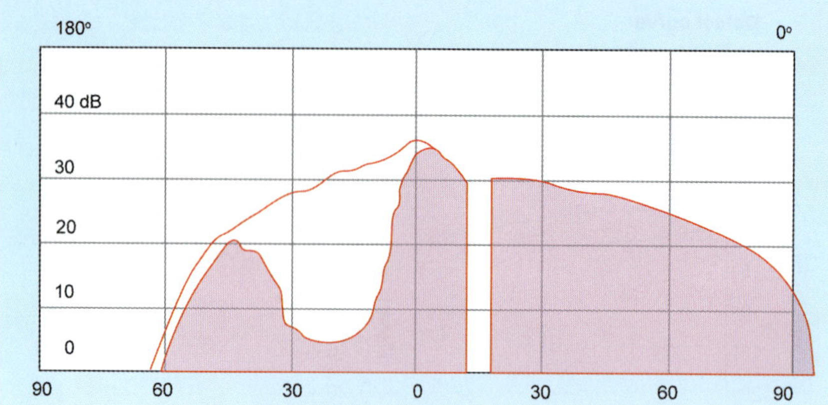

Fig. 39: High deviation (LV/ PSD).

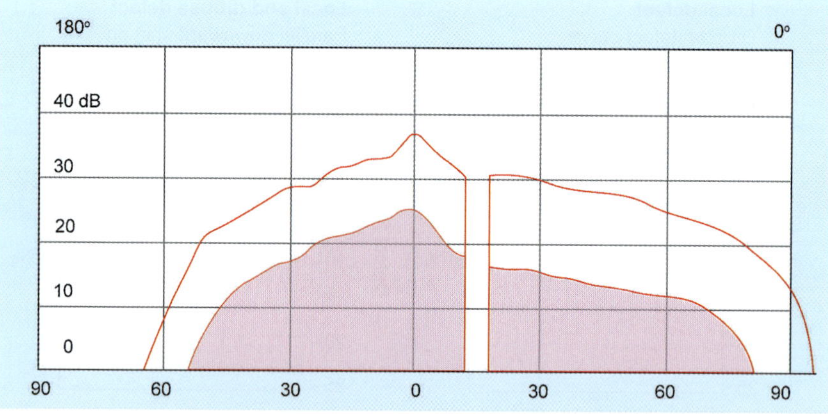

Fig. 40: Low LV/PSD. (LV/PSD: local visual/pattern standard deviation)

by the retinal nerve fiber bundles in the retina. The cluster analysis displays 10 visual field clusters that spatially correlate with retinal nerve fiber bundles. In each cluster, the average sensitivity loss is calculated and presented as a cluster MD **(Figs. 41A and B)**.

From the cluster analysis, another parameter called the collected cluster analysis is calculated. It is the arithmetic mean of all defects within one cluster which results in the cluster MD. The concept of probabilities as presented in the probabilities representation is as follows **(Fig. 42)**:

- P > 5%: +, P 1–5%: unbold font, P < **1%**: **bold font**
- *Polar analysis* ***(Fig. 43)***

Trend analysis: The trend analysis of global indices such as MD or sLV takes into consideration loss in sensitivity due to cataract also in follow up analysis Gray line—normal values, Red line: 15 dB mark for highlighting worsening of quality of vision **(Figs. 44 to 47).**

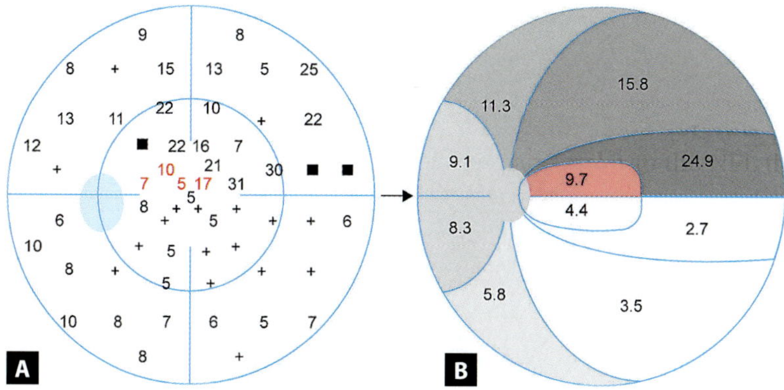

Figs. 41A and B: Cluster analysis.

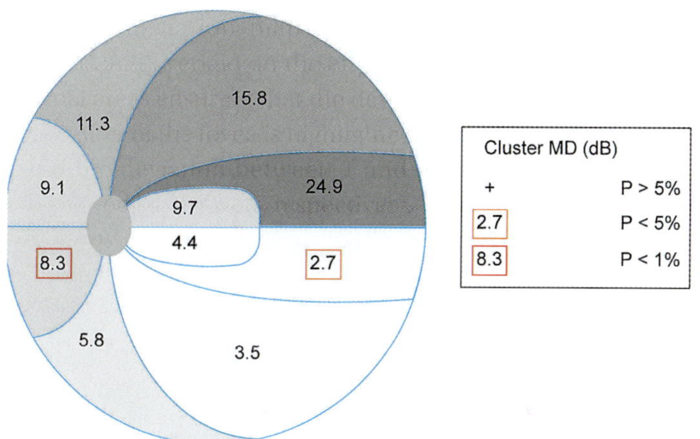

Fig. 42: Cluster MD with probability.

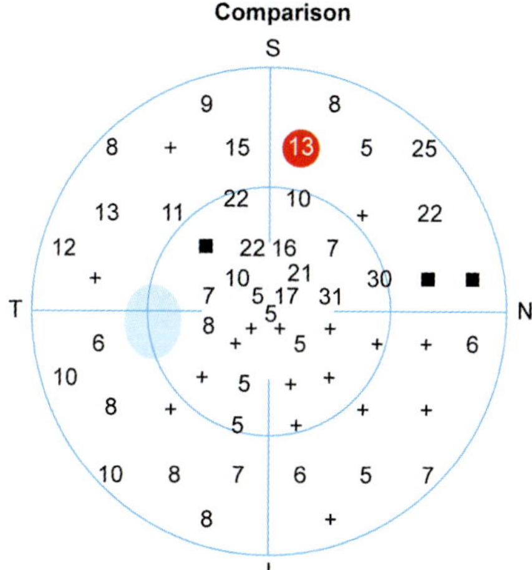

Fig. 43: Polar analysis.

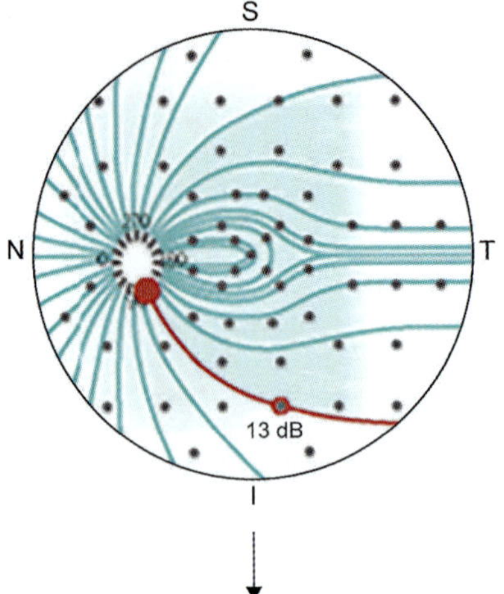

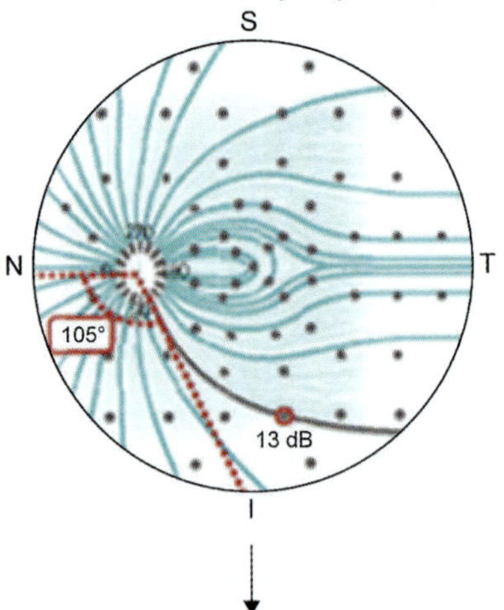

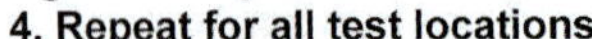

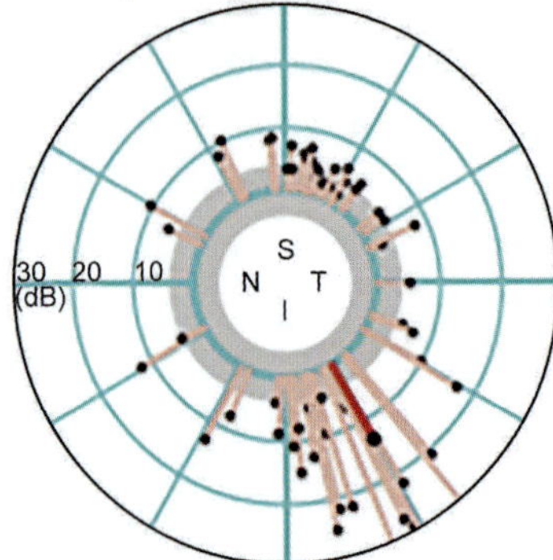

Fig. 44: Polar trends highlighting worsening of quality of vision.

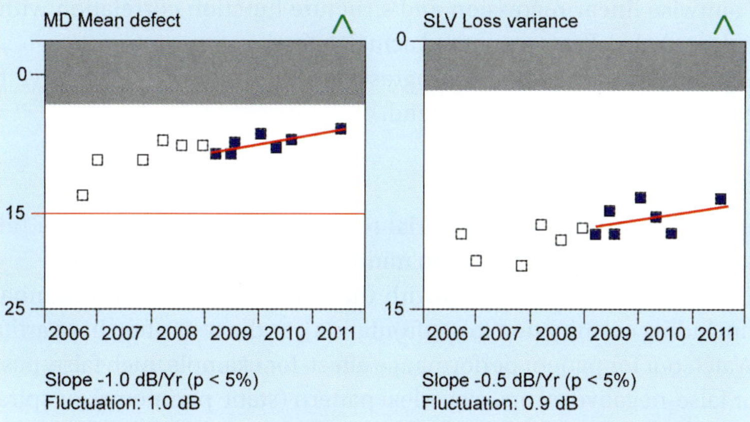

Fig. 45: Change in mean defect and Square of loss of variance (sLV) over a period of time.

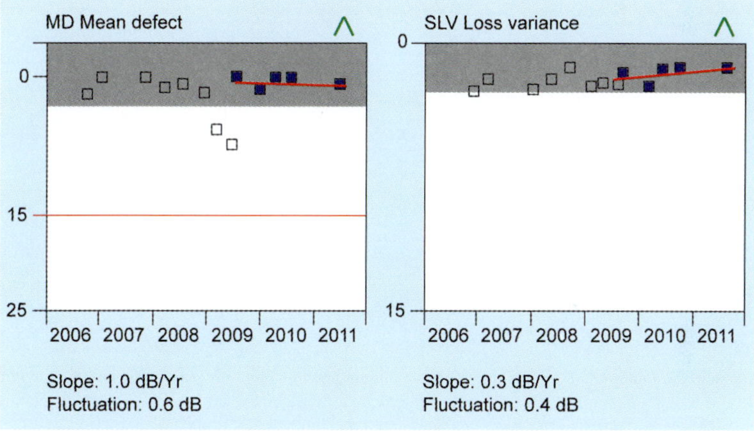

Fig. 46: showspolar trends and cluster trends in looking at progression.

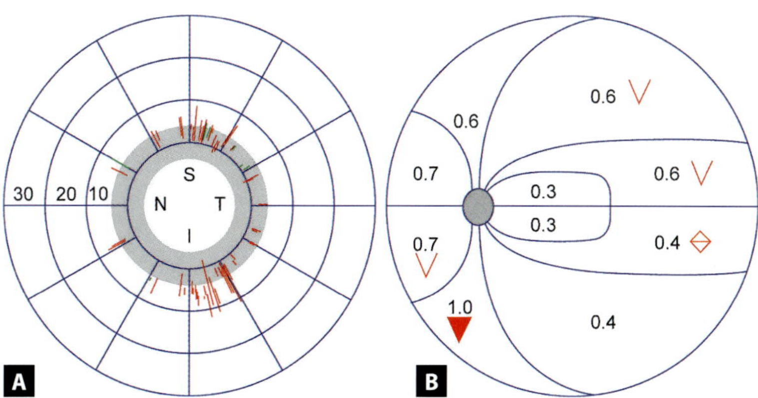

Figs. 47A and B: (A) Polar trend and (B) Cluster trend.

- Pointwise linear regression and structure function correlation with the polar trend (reflects smoothed actual defect).
- Significance of trend and progression rate in dB/year per nerve fiber cluster is seen in the cluster trend.

TO SUMMARIZE

- Perimetry results give a pictorial representation of the patient's "hill of vision"; keep the normal hill in mind when reviewing these tests.
- Correlate perimetry results with the clinical history and examination (including examination to confrontation), as the tests often have artifacts.
- Watch out for patient performance effect, for example, high false-positive or false-negative errors, cloverleaf pattern (static perimetry), or spiraling of fields (kinetic fields).
- Static and kinetic perimetry complement one another; consider the other if the first is unexpectedly normal or abnormal.

CHAPTER

Imaging in Ophthalmology

Sachin S Dharwadkar

INTRODUCTION

Imaging in ophthalmology has come of age especially in relation to glaucoma.

Glaucoma as we also know is a progressive and irreversible disease in most and the Holy Grail lies in identifying and arresting progression to visual handicap.

The visual field test being a subjective test plagued by a long testing time and a high test-retest variability in a significant amount of those tested. It has found a good companion in optical coherence tomography (OCT) to aid our decision making in glaucoma cases. Being fully objective and fast, OCT becomes a great asset.

It is of great importance to note that many times the OCT measurements and clinical impression of fundus also may differ greatly which makes imaging very invaluable.

The transition from Heidelberg Retina Tomograph (HRT), GDx, and the primitive OCT of the yesteryears has now finally given way to a technology that can by and large measure the optic nerve head and posterior pole with a minimal inter-test variations if done diligently.

The modern-day OCT can measure the ganglion cell to the axonal exit at the optic nerve head in its entirety and give us an estimate of nerve health in the individual tested. The measured parameters that are available to us vary with the machine made in consideration. From the physics standpoint, the current OCTs are divided into the swept-source and the spectral domain OCT differentiated basis of the used light source.

The spectral domain OCTs give a better resolution whereas the swept source in general measures deeper and over a larger area at the cost of resolution.

Examples of the swept-source OCT are the TRITON from Topcon and Spectralis and Cirrus are examples of the spectral domain OCTs.

The parameters that merit consideration in OCT (from a glaucoma standpoint) are the disc area, rim width, retinal nerve fiber layer (RNFL) thickness, and macular ganglion cell thickness. All these parameters need simultaneous consideration, and one should desist using them separately or comparing efficacy of one parameter over the other for glaucoma assessment.

Some machines provide a cup-to-disc (CD) ratio and other measures that are not strictly correlated to the visualized disc parameters on clinical biomicroscopic fundus examination due to the assumptions involved in their calculations.

It is recommended that a thorough knowledge of physics and functioning of the machine is essential before one uses OCT for clinical decision making. Using OCT in glaucoma is not just as simple as looking at/interpreting the reports.

Poor understanding and not using appropriate checklists can result in potential abuse of this technology causing more harm than good.

Some important aspects of OCT in glaucoma are as follows:

- Standardization of image quality with appropriate and standard acquisition protocols.
- Using machines having hardware that can help to reduce test-retest variability by scanning the same locations as in the baseline all the time.
- Normative database in the used machine that is representative of the population examined.
- Images that can be edited if necessary and errors observed.
- *Machines that give all aspects:* Disc, RNFL, macula, and/or subcomponent scans—ganglion cell layer (GCL), ganglion cell-inner plexiform layer (GC-IPL), and ganglion cell complex (GCC) in one report.

Once the images are obtained of an acceptable standard (image quality criteria differ as per machine used) then the process of interpretation can start.

However, it is to be noted that these tests help to confirm a diagnosis rather than make one. Diagnosis is the clinician's responsibility.

NORMATIVE DATA CONUNDRUM

- Normative data is the data that is of age and gender-matched "normal" population.
- It is highly dependent on the population examined while generating the database and always limited in its scope and applicability.
- It cannot be all encompassing and cannot account for all anatomical and structural variations.
- Even when the populace is the same there can be wide spectrum of "normal" that can be "flagged".
- Thus, it can be considered at the best guideline/supportive evidence and not a confirmation of disease.
- The statistical meaning of the deviations from normative data has to be understood well and color codes are not to be taken as pointers of pathology (genesis of red and green disease)

Example: For Cirrus high-definition (HD) OCT, the normative data is for 282 individuals above the age of 18 years in a certain range of refractive error (-12 to +6) for this machine. Suffice to say this cannot be in any way representative of even a fraction of permutations in the world.

Besides, the assumption is that the measurements in the normative data are presumed to have normal distribution.

Thus, before the color is given any importance to the suspected area of pathology, the correlation with area of the map that is flagged is of cardinal importance in diagnosis.

The most foolproof way of using OCT for glaucoma is using it for progression assessment with patients' own data as baseline and "normative" at time of presentation. The caveat though is that the tracking system of the machine has to be extremely robust and foolproof.

GENERIC STEPS IN INTERPRETING OPTICAL COHERENCE TOMOGRAPHY SCAN

- Considering the commonly used Cirrus scan as a prototype
- All the images in the tomogram maps are preferably to be in monochrome to aid proper assessment.

Retinal nerve fiber layer OU map and ganglion cell OU printout to be considered together as a rule. Summary of these two can be provided as PanoMap to patients. Clinicians should however have both these maps as they contain the tomograms necessary for the necessary image audits before interpreting.

Retinal Nerve Fiber Layer OU Map

- *Patient data:* At top of all maps it is important to verify patient details.
- *Checking image quality:* Checked at three places (1) image score given by machine: should be as per manufacturer recommendation or maximum possible, (2) thickness map for black spots and RNFL deviation map for disc—frame shift artifacts, and (3) tomography maps: check segmentation lines (better in monochrome).
- RNFL thickness map is color-coded map (legend on side, cool meaning thinner) for representing thickness distribution of nerve fiber layer (NFL) in a given patient. This map can be considered "raw distribution" unrelated to normative data. Usage of false color in this map is intuitive in finding areas of thinning and any abnormal patterns of distribution of NFL.
- *RNFL deviation map:* It is placed below the thickness map. This is the comparison to the normative data. It shows an en-face infrared reflectance (IR) image with a superimposed scanning/calculation circle—purple, BMO border—black, and cup border—red. As name suggests, this is

comparison to the normative database and is represented as colored superpixels to aid interpretation. At <5% (percentile) of normative data shown as yellow and at <1% shown as red superpixels. The only difference for models more advanced than the Cirrus 500 is that the outlines of the map would be of green/blue lines indicating tracking system usage.

- *Key parameters table:* After the verification and due diligence on examination quality and qualitative distribution of thickness data, attention can be shifted to numerical values of parameters table. All seven parameters are compared to the normative data and color-coded. Gray—outside database, and red, yellow, green for values <1%, 1–5%, and 5–95%, respectively and white >95%.
- *Neuroretinal rim thickness plot:* In temporal-superior-nasal-inferior-temporal (TSNIT) configuration, it is measured between the red (cup) and black (BMO) and compared age and disc size matched to normative data and represented on color-coded TSNIT curve.
- *RNFL thickness TSNIT plot:* Calculated at the 3.46 mm distance from BMO center (automated identification in newer machines which is the way to go as BMO cannot be identified by naked eye). Patients RNFL data are plotted against age-matched normative data as for the neuroretinal rim. Usually, they have a double hump configuration if normal and it is important here to note intereye asymmetry besides comparison with the normative data.
- *Quadrant and sector-wise RNFL data:* Sector-wise classification of the NFL data basis distribution of normal scale that helps in identification of local changes and remove averaging effect of quadrantic representation. Clinical correlation with fundus examination is solicited here.

Ganglion Cell Map

In Cirrus, this map is calculated using the 512 × 128 scan grid in a 6 × 6 mm cube centered on fovea.

The art of reading the report is similar to the pattern followed for all OCT reports that starts from scan quality and patient data and due diligence on the segmented images before observing actual values and intereye asymmetry.

As in the disc NFL printout, simple steps are as follows:

1. *Quality and patient data:*
    - To verify patient details and scan score. Quality yardsticks same as RNFL scan and the horizontal B scan—segmented image
    - At the bottom, it should be inspected in gray scale at this stage to look for errors. In case of errors here, the report has to be discarded irrespective of scan score.

2. *Thickness map:* It measures the segmented GC-IPL (proprietary to Zeiss machine) in the 6 × 6 mm cube already mentioned.

   The normal shape expected is an elliptical horizontal annulus centered on the fovea. Thickness scale/color code for this "raw measurement" is shown on the left of the map similar to the NFL thickness map.

   The important part at this stage is to verify placement and centration of the annulus on the fovea (that has been detected by automated methods) to prevent the occurrence of artifacts.

   The points to note here are black shading on maps for shadowing artifacts (indicate poor scan quality), the focal notches in the annulus, and intereye asymmetry of the macular maps.
3. *Deviation maps:* Comparing the acquired raw data to age-matched normal, the deviation map is generated in forms of color-coded superpixels and overlaid on the en face IR macula image. No color code for normal areas ensuring that the deviations are highlighted.

   The center of the fovea is highlighted with a purple oval for identification and the deviation between 1 and 5% and <1% are highlighted in yellow and red superpixels, respectively.
4. *Sector maps:* Measurements are provided in the annulus between 1.2 × 1 mm and 4.8 × 4 mm around the center of fovea where the GC-IPL is the most prominent, divided into three mirrored symmetric regions superiorly and inferiorly with reference to horizontal midline. These maps are color coded as per the color code legend provided to indicate statistical significance as in other maps.
5. *Thickness table:* It shows average and minimum GC-IPL measurements; it is a snapshot comparison of both eyes in numerical values.

   Besides these maps, combination prints that include the optic nerve head (ONH), NFL, GC-IPL like PanoMaps, etc. (Zeiss and Cirrus) are available that can be used to explain the patients or as a teaching tool.

   What is important though is that the patient should also carry a report that has a tomogram incorporated for proper due diligence (not available in PanoMap representation).

PROGRESSION ANALYSIS ON OPTICAL COHERENCE TOMOGRAPHY

This is the Holy Grail of OCT usage in glaucoma assessment and monitoring.

- Unfortunately, all machines available are not capable or equipped for doing this effectively and in a foolproof manner.
- The basis requirement for this aspect is ultrafast scanning protocols and an equally good tracking system.

- It will also help if the machine allows image auditing/editing capability and multiple imaging safeguards incorporated.

Let us discuss progression assessment in relation to the Cirrus OCT machine:

Patient data, scan parameters (quality, segmentation, alignment, and acquisition)—proprietary quality score as per recommendation, segmentation artifacts due to pathology (CME, PVD, etc.) in each scan selected. Signal strength and artifacts (black spots in the thickness maps on printout—Cirrus)

- Check for the alignment method in each follow-up scan (R2—in Cirrus) to ensure appropriateness of the images used for analysis
- Look at the event and trend analysis printout. In the event analysis, the thickness and change maps are available in the Cirrus.
- If the change exceeds the test-retest variability the region is marked in yellow and brown superpixels.
- Another part of the event map in Cirrus is the RNFL thickness profile change map. Current examination compared with baseline and presented as a superimposition and changes flagged in color code mentioned as legend.
- The trend analysis is represented by linear regression of CD ratio, and Avg, superior and inferior NFL thickness averages plotted over time. The rate values therein give an idea for clinical significance. Any outlier in this map is a red flag and a subtle suggestion to visit scan on the console.
- *RNFL and ONH progression summary:* Summarizes the parameters into a simple color-coded representation
- Important labels are "possible loss" and "likely loss" when change exceeds test-retest variability on one or multiple occasions. "Possible increase" only occurs due to artifact or pathology such as traction or edema.
- Outliers in imaging are red flags that need revision or exclusion.
- If due diligence is proper and SOPs for imaging are in place, using the right machines can surely be instrumental in taking use of imaging in glaucoma progression to the next level.

Thus, the use of imaging in glaucoma progression is one that has come to stay and will only get better with new innovations in time. Understanding machine physics and strict checklist adoptions will go a great way in helping us tide over the test-retest variability of perimetry in many of the indicated cases.

CHAPTER

Primary Congenital Glaucoma

Vyshak AS, Anchal Gera, Sushmita Kaushik

INTRODUCTION

Primary congenital glaucoma (PCG) is a major cause of childhood visual dysfunction. It occurs due to maldevelopment of the trabecular meshwork (TM) and anterior chamber (AC) angle, which prevents proper drainage of aqueous humor. PCG is typically noticed at birth or early childhood and is not associated with other ocular or systemic abnormalities. Its early onset and significant impact on patients' future quality of life raise concerns about this childhood condition.

The prevalence of PCG varies among races, geographic regions, and the frequency of consanguinity. It lies in 1 per 10,000 live births in Western countries, 1:3,300 in Andhra Pradesh in India, 1:2,500 in Middle East countries, and the highest of 1:1,250 in Gypsy of Slovakia.

For a better understanding of PCG, more insights into the etiology, pathogenesis, clinical characteristics, and treatment are essential.

ETIOLOGY AND PATHOGENESIS

Genetic Mutations

As a primary congenital disorder, it is estimated that 10–40% of PCG patients are familial and show autosomal recessive inheritance patterns. Several genes at different loci have been reported, among which the three most well-known implicated genes are cytochrome P450 family 1 subfamily B polypeptide 1 (*CYP1B1*) located in the 2p21 (GLC3A), latent transforming growth factor β-binding protein 2 (*LTBP2*) located at 14q24 (GLC3D), and myocilin (*MYOC*). Another recently reported protein product was Angio protein receptor tunica interna endothelial cell kinase (TEK) encoded by the *TEK* gene. Given that the functions of protein products vary, the underlying genetic mechanisms involved in PCG could, to some extent, be explained by the dysfunctional proteins that interfere with either the outflow pathway (specifically the TM or the Schlemm's canal).

Among all the genes mentioned above, *CYP1B1* is the most frequent cause of PCG worldwide, as 20–90% of familial PCG cases and up to 27% of sporadic cases map to this gene. The patients with *CYP1B1* mutations tended to have an earlier onset age and worse outcomes after surgery.

The clinical significance of recognizing the role of these genes paves the way for the early diagnosis and future development of gene therapies in PCG.

PATHOGENESIS OF PRIMARY CONGENITAL GLAUCOMA: THEORIES AND HYPOTHESES

Although it is widely acknowledged that angle structure malformation and congenital AC angle dysplasia were culprits for PCG, the exact pathogenesis of PCG remains unclear.

After observing the shiny appearance and subsequent falling back of the peripheral iris following goniotomy, Barkan suggested that an anatomical abnormality, a "pseudomembrane", obstructs the outflow of aqueous humor due to a high iris insertion. This led to the introduction of goniotomy in 1938, which significantly improved the poor prognosis of PCG. However, detailed histologic studies have not confirmed the existence of this "impermeable membrane". Other researchers have suggested that the observed "membrane" is compacted trabecular sheets, preventing the visualization of the normal posterior recess of the ciliary body and iris.

Compared with the membrane theory from the perspective of histomorphology, the role of neural crest cells has been highly appreciated. It is understood that angle structures primarily originate from neural crest cells. This has led to the hypothesis that the immature angle appearance and drainage angle anomaly in PCG may be attributed to the developmental arrest of neural crest cells in the third trimester. Additionally, others have suggested that defects in the gene expression of neural crest cells also play a role.

Additionally, there are other less noticeable theories, such as the contraction or separation of the angle and ciliary body pushing the TM. The latter is indirectly supported by angle surgeries that work by changing the relationship between the ciliary muscle and the TM. It is important to note that all of the aforementioned theories ultimately relate to trabeculodysgenesis, leading to PCG.

CLINICAL CHARACTERISTICS OF PRIMARY CONGENITAL GLAUCOMA

According to the European Glaucoma Society Terminology and Guidelines for Glaucoma (5th edition), PCG can be categorized into three subtypes based on the age of onset:

1. *Neonatal onset PCG:* Elevated intraocular pressure (IOP) present in the womb or diagnosed within the first month of life.
2. *Infantile-onset PCG:* It occurs between 1 and 24 months after birth.

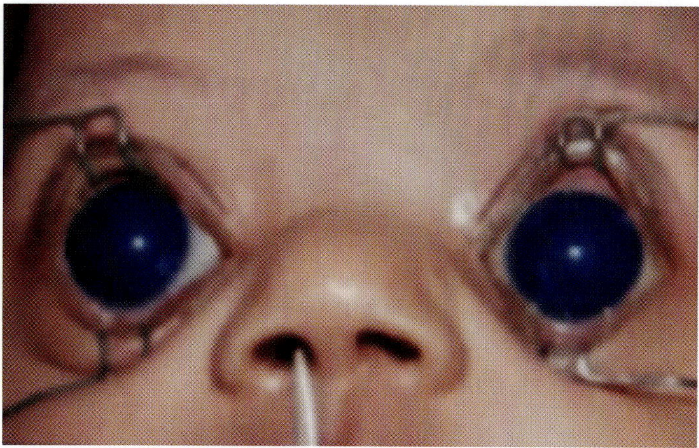

Fig. 1: Primary congenital glaucoma presenting with enlarged eyeballs and cloudy corneas.

3. *Late-onset PCG:* Elevated IOP with evidence of buphthalmos, diagnosed from age of 2 years to puberty.

This classification serves as the foundation for clinical diagnosis, treatment decisions, and long-term prognosis of PCG.

Primary congenital glaucoma occurring in infancy commonly presents with one or more of the classic triad of photophobia, epiphora, and blepharospasm though they commonly give a first impression of an enlarged eyeball (buphthalmos). Other signs of PCG include corneal opacity, increased corneal diameter, horizontal or sometimes circumferential breaks of the Descemet membrane (Haab's striae), elevated IOP, and optic disc excavation. Neonatal-onset glaucoma often presents with a cloudy cornea at birth **(Fig. 1)**.

The gender ratio of PCG showed a male preponderance. The manifestation can be unilateral or asymmetrically bilateral, yet bilateral cases dominate with a proportion of 65–75%, especially among those with *CYP1B1* mutation.

DIFFERENTIAL DIAGNOSIS

The three pillars of PCG diagnosis are photophobia, lacrimation, and blepharospasm, commonly associated with buphthalmos (enlarged eyeballs) and variable corneal clarity **(Figs. 2A and B)**.

Some of these are also found in other conditions.

Excessive tearing: Congenital nasolacrimal duct obstruction, conjunctivitis, corneal injury, or keratitis.

Large corneas: Congenital megalocornea—X-linked recessive disorder with bilaterally enlarged corneas, normal IOP, and cup-disc ratio.

Axial myopia also has enlarged eyeballs with normal IOP and the optic disc, but myopic fundus gives a clue.

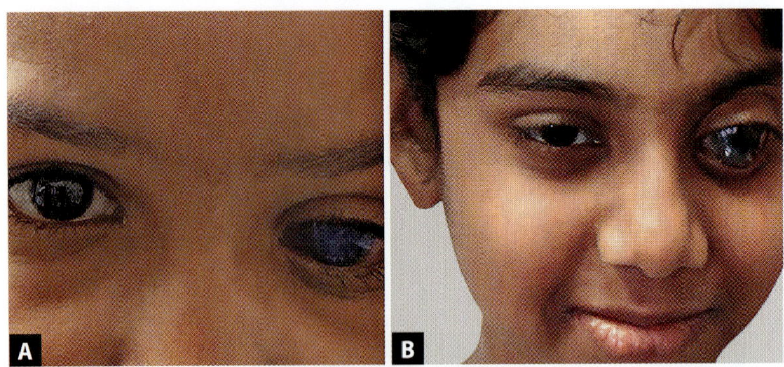

Figs. 2A and B: Left eye buphthalmos.

Corneal opacification: Refer to mnemonic STUMPED—
S: Sclerocornea
T: Trauma, tears in Descemet membrane
U: Ulcers in the cornea
M: Metabolic disorders
P: Peters anomaly
E: Endothelial dystrophy
D: Dermoid

Primary congenital glaucoma is considered a subset of anterior segment dysgenesis where only isolated trabeculodysgenesis or goniodysgenesis occurs.

The differential diagnosis of PCG must include other childhood glaucomas, especially those with nonacquired ocular anomalies. When there are associated ocular and facial abnormalities mostly of neural crest cell origin such as TM, iris, and cornea, they are denoted as developmental glaucoma or glaucoma associated with nonacquired ocular anomalies as per classification by Childhood Glaucoma Research Network (CGRN).

Glaucoma Associated with Nonacquired Ocular Anomalies

Axenfeld–Rieger Syndrome

Axenfeld-Rieger syndrome (ARS) is a group of autosomal dominant disorders with high penetrance and variable expressivity. Traditionally, ARS is subdivided into: (1) Axenfeld anomaly (peripheral anterior segment anomalies such as posterior embryotoxon), (2) anomaly (mesodermal dysgenesis of iris and cornea such as polycoria and corectopia), (3) ARS (ocular anomalies with systemic developmental defects of teeth and bones microdontia, hypodontia, oligodontia, hypertelorism, telecanthus, broad flat nose, micrognathia, mandibular prognathism, hypospadias, pituitary abnormalities, and umbilical abnormalities).

Now, these ocular findings and associated systemic manifestations are recognized under ARS.

Peters Anomaly

Peters presents with early-onset buphthalmos and central corneal opacities, mostly bilaterally. Most cases are sporadic, but autosomal recessive and less commonly autosomal dominant inheritance have been described, caused by mutations in *PAX6, PITX2, CYP1B1,* or *FOXC1* gene.

It is subgrouped into three types:

Peters 1: Hallmark is the central corneal abnormality as a result of a variable defect in the Descemet membrane and corneal endothelium with associated iridocorneal synechia.

Peters 2: All features of Peters 1 with additional features of lens abnormalities, commonly corner-lenticular adhesions and cataracts.

Peters plus syndrome: Systemic abnormalities such as short stature, developmental delay, dysmorphic facial features, cardiac, genitourinary, and central nervous system abnormalities.

Aniridia

Aniridia is a rare genetic disorder with variable degrees of iris hypoplasia or absence of iris commonly associated with early-onset foveal hypoplasia, reduced visual acuity, and nystagmus.

Frequently also presents with limbal stem cell deficiency, glaucoma, and cataracts.

Two-thirds of cases have autosomal dominant inheritance, one-third are sporadic, and both involve mutations in the *PAX6* gene and its regulatory regions. Large deletions may extend to involve adjacent *WT1* genes, resulting in WAGR syndrome. 2% are of autosomal recessive inheritance, also known as Gillespie syndrome. It is associated with cerebellar ataxia and intellectual disability.

Initially, the angle is open, which gets covered with the rudimentary iris tissue stump over time. Glaucoma develops in 50–75% of aniridia patients, usually around late childhood, due to abnormal angle development. Anterior rotation of the ciliary body is also hypothesized to have a role. When glaucoma presents early, it is likely due to congenital anomalies in the filtration angle.

Neonatal-onset Congenital Ectropion Uvea

Neonatal-onset congenital ectropion uvea (N-CEU) presents with early onset severe, intractable glaucoma with bilateral buphthalmos, central spindle-shaped corneal opacities, deep AC, featureless angle, and ectropion uvea. They present with homozygous mutations in the *CYP1B1* gene change of protein Arg390His.

MANAGEMENT

Medical Therapy

The cause of raised IOP is a developmental anomaly of the angle structures, which requires surgical intervention as a definitive measure, in the meantime, the child is started on antiglaucoma medications to clear the cornea and buy time till preanesthetic clearances and systemic evaluations are completed. IOP in a normal infant is 8–12 mm Hg and 10–14 mm Hg in adolescent children. It is safe to start treatment with topical carbonic anhydrase inhibitors and β-blockers. If required, prostaglandin analogs can be added. α-receptor blocking aqueous suppressing agents such as brimonidine are avoided in children <6 years or 20 kg weight. They are known to cause central nervous system (CNS) depression, fatigue, and respiratory center depression due to their ability to cross the brain barrier. Oral carbonic anhydrase inhibitors can be added if required with a dosing of 15 mg/kg/day in three divided doses.

Surgical Management

Surgical management aims to primarily increase the outflow or, as a last resort, decrease the production of aqueous. Choice of surgery depends on the severity of glaucoma, cornea clarity (angle visibility), surgeon's expertise, and affordability. Often, repeat surgeries may be required.

Surgeries to increase outflow include:

Angle Procedures

When the angle can be seen under direct visualization, and the disease is not severe, a goniotomy can be done to treat the nasal angle in an ab-interno approach where the TM beams can be simply cut with a microvitreoretinal (MVR) blade. If the cornea is not clear, then trabeculotomy is done in an ab-externo approach, here, a limbus-based conjunctival flap is fashioned, followed by a partial thickness scleral flap. A scleral incision is made, and the Schlemm canal is exposed. Harms trabeculotome is passed along the canal, and the inner prongs are used to break the inner wall of the canal in both directions. This can be used to treat 120–180° of the angle. A 360° trabeculotomy can be performed using an illuminated cannula passed through the AC.

Filtration Procedures

Trabeculectomy alone or in adjunct with mitomycin C (MMC) or a glaucoma drainage device (GDD) can be placed. Trabeculectomy alone is usually not preferred in children due to increased healing response, early fibrosis, and failure of the bleb. The use of mitomycin can cause thinning of epithelium with the development of thin avascular blebs, which may predispose to bleb leaks and blebitis. The success rate ranges between 60 and 65%.

Deep sclerectomy: It involves creation of a partial thickness scleral flap and removal of the external portion of scheme canal and TM.

Glaucoma drainage devices are mostly reserved for refractory cases where primary angle procedures have failed, as they are commonly associated with endothelial loss and corneal decompensation, resulting in loss of vision.

Combined Trabeculotomy with Trabeculectomy

A combined trabeculotomy with trabeculectomy (CTT) with or without MMC is commonly the surgery of choice in cases of severe glaucoma, corneal opacity with poor angle visibility, or failed angle surgery. A limbus-based conjunctival flap is raised, followed by a 4 × 4 mm scleral flap. MMC in strength of 0.02/0.04% is applied for 1–4 minutes duration followed by a radial incision to reach the Schlemm canal, trabeculotomy is done with Harms trabeculotome. A full-thickness scleral ostium is excised (1–3 mm), followed by completion of surgical iridectomy. The scleral flap is sutured with 10-0 monofilament nylon suture, and the conjunctiva is closed with 8-0 Vicryl suture.

Cyclodestructive Procedures

Cyclodestructive procedures decrease aqueous production by destroying the secretory ciliary epithelium. The ciliary epithelium can regenerate. Hence, multiple treatments may be necessary.

Commonly, diode laser photocoagulation is delivered via the ab-externo route by diode laser cyclophotocoagulation (DLCP) and Micropulse laser therapy or under direct visualization by endocyclophotocoagulation. This procedure is reserved for refractory cases with poor or nil visual prognosis.

PROGNOSIS

The prognosis is variable. If left untreated, PCG almost always leads to blindness and buphthalmos with variable degrees of corneal opacity and optic nerve head damage. Early presentation—neonatal-onset PCG usually indicates severe angle structure abnormalities and tends to perform worse compared to infantile-onset PCG in terms of IOP control and surgical success. In general, IOP control is achieved in 80% of PCG children.

Children with infantile-onset PCG presenting early with prompt surgical intervention have the best prognosis for IOP control and visual rehabilitation.

The prognosis is ongoing, and children with PCG require regular examinations under anesthesia (EUA) every 3–4 months postsurgery for a year, then 6 months till the child is cooperative enough for thorough clinical examination, usually achieved by 5 years of age.

Lifelong follow-up must be explained to the patient's family.

VISUAL REHABILITATION

Only 35% of all patients have visual acuity better than 6/15 on Snellen's, and 2–15% of childhood glaucoma children become blind.

Visual prognosis depends on baseline optic nerve head damage, corneal opacification, ongoing IOP control, status of concomitant anterior and posterior segment anomalies, strabismus, and amblyopia.

In children with corneal opacities obscuring the visual axis, inferior optical iridectomies must be performed early to avoid amblyopia while the child awaits corneal transplant surgery.

In children with clear visual axis, effort must be made to have cycloplegic refraction as per age in phakic children and dry refraction for pseudophakic and aphakic children with appropriate near add corrections and prescription of executive bifocals in all EUAs or at least 6 monthly.

Patching of the better eye must be offered to all children with the best refractive error correction to reduce amblyopia.

Disclosure: There are no financial disclosures.

SUGGESTED READING

1. Aktas Z, Ucgul AY, Ikiz GD. Glaucoma Associated with Non-acquired Ocular Disorders. In: El Sayed YM, Elhusseiny AM (Eds). Childhood Glaucoma. Cham: Springer; 2024.
2. Al-Shahwan S, Al-Torbak AA, Turkmani S, Al-Omran M, Al-Jadaan I, Edward DP. Side-effect profile of brimonidine tartrate in children. Ophthalmology. 2005;112(12):2143.
3. Badawi AH, Al-Muhaylib AA, Al Owaifeer AM, Al-Essa RS, Al-Shahwan SA. Primary congenital glaucoma: An updated review. Saudi J Ophthalmol. 2019;33:382-8.
4. Dandona L, Williams JD, Williams BC, Rao GN. Population-based assessment of childhood blindness in southern India. Arch Ophthalmol. 1998;116(4):545-6.
5. Gage PJ, Rhoades W, Prucka SK, Hjalt T. Fate maps of neural crest and mesoderm in the mammalian eye. Invest Ophthalmol Vis Sci. 2005;46:4200-8.
6. Gupta V, Jha R, Srinivasan G, Dada T, Sihota R. Ultrasound biomicroscopic characteristics of the anterior segment in primary congenital glaucoma. J AAPOS. 2007;11:546-50.
7. Kaushik S, Dhingra D, Vibha B, Saini A, Gupta G, Snehi S, et al. Neonatal-Onset Congenital Ectropion Uveae: A Distinct Phenotype of Newborn Glaucoma. Am J Ophthalmol. 2021;223:83-90.
8. Mocan MC, Mehta AA, Aref AA. Update in genetics and surgical management of primary congenital glaucoma. Turk J Ophthalmol. 2019;49:347-55.
9. Shaffer RN. Prognosis of goniotomy in primary infantile glaucoma (trabeculodysgenesis). Trans Am Ophthalmol Soc. 1982;80:321-5.
10. Souma T, Tompson SW, Thomson BR, Siggs OM, Kizhatil K, Yamaguchi S, et al. Angiopoietin receptor TEK mutations underlie primary congenital glaucoma with variable expressivity. J Clin Invest. 2016;126:2575-87.
11. Thau A, Lloyd M, Freedman S, Beck A, Grajewski A, Levin AV. New classification system for pediatric glaucoma: implications for clinical care and a research registry. Curr Opin Ophthalmol. 2018;29(5):385-394.

CHAPTER 8

Primary Angle-closure Glaucoma

Meenakshi Y Dhar

INTRODUCTION

- Glaucoma is a progressive optic neuropathy with characteristic changes in the optic nerve head (ONH) and visual fields where intraocular pressure (IOP) is only a modifiable factor. Primary glaucomas occur without any external cause of two types: (1) primary open-angle glaucoma (POAG) or primary angle-closure glaucoma (PACG).
- Primary angle-closure disease (PACD) is the form of glaucoma characterized by narrowing or closure of the anterior chamber (AC) angle with contact between iris and trabecular meshwork, leading to impaired outflow of aqueous humor mechanically, raises IOP, damages the optic nerve irreversibly and leads to loss of vision if untreated. It is a serious and potentially blinding condition. Angle closure is an ongoing process.
- The angle closure occurs primarily due to anatomical factors and not due to secondary causes such as trauma or inflammation. Gonioscopy done in a dark room with a 1-mm slit beam clinches the diagnosis. Nonvisibility of posterior pigmented trabecular meshwork in 180° or greater of the angle circumference in the primary position is defined as an *occludable angle*. PACD is a spectrum—on the one hand there is an asymptomatic patient with narrow angles, normal IOP, and normal visual function; and on the other hand, there are patients with narrow angles and raised IOP, with/without symptoms (blurring/intermittent pain), ± visual field defects, having characteristic ONH changes of glaucoma, which may eventually lead to loss of vision and blindness. Infrequently, it presents as an emergency with sudden rise in IOP, having acute symptoms of pain, visual loss, headache, and vomiting requiring urgent management. Most often PACD is insidious, chronic, and asymptomatic. The glaucoma continuum given by Weinreb et al. for POAG can even be applied to patients of PACG other than the acute attack to explain it to patients with certain changes. PACG has been shown to have higher IOPs than POAG and progresses faster to blindness. In contrast to POAG, long-term clinically applicable algorithms of PACG are few, and even those available are not being followed by most clinicians. Laser peripheral iridotomy (LPI) can favorably change the course of the disease.

CLASSIFICATION

There have been different classifications of angle-closure disease—primary angle closure (PAC) is a spectrum with a similar pathology and the entire gamut could be designated "primary angle-closure disease (PACD)". The current classification of PACG was given by International Society for Geographical and Epidemiological Ophthalmology (ISGEO) is based on natural history of the disease.

- *Primary angle-closure suspect (PACS):* ≥180° iridotrabecular contact (ITC), normal IOP, and no ONH damage and normal visual fields
- *PAC:* ≥180° ITC with peripheral anterior synechiae (PAS) or elevated IOP but no optic neuropathy.
- *PACG:* ≥180° ITC with PAS, elevated IOP, and glaucomatous optic neuropathy (GON) and typical visual fields defects. Severity is classified as mild, moderate, and severe based on Hodapp-Parrish-Anderson criteria.

1 in 4 will progress from PACS to PAC over 5 years, and the same is for progression from PAC to PACG. Progression is more likely to occur in those bilateral PACS, PAC with OHT, and those without LPI. Some PAC will have GON, high IOP but only appositional closure—they are the mixed form with both open-angle and angle-closure mechanism at play.

- *Acute angle-closure glaucoma (AACG):* Occluded angle with symptomatic high IOP
- *Plateau iris configuration:* Narrow angle due to an anteriorly positioned ciliary body, with deep central AC.
- *Plateau iris syndrome:* Narrow angle due to an anteriorly positioned ciliary body with deep central AC, and any ITC persisting after patent peripheral iridotomy

EPIDEMIOLOGY

Prevalence: PACG is more common in certain ethnic groups, particularly in people of East Asian descent and Indians. It is the leading cause of blindness in Asia.

In India, it may be as prevalent as POAG. PACG is a more blinding disease than POAG and blindness in those with PACG are twice as often bilaterally blind. Surgical intervention is needed more often in PACG. 2.54 million Indians have PACG and 0.25 million are blind due to PACG as per deductions from the few scattered population studies that are published from India in 2018.

It has a preponderance in women, especially in the middle age (above 50 years of age). In a study done by Das et al. in North India, male: female ratio was 48.6:51.4. Women predominated in those with acute presentation AACG (79.8%) and subacute PAC (66.7%) while males had chronic PACG (75.4%).

The risk of PACD increases with age and it generally occurs after 40 years of age. AACG manifests it in the third and fourth decade, while subacute PAC in the fourth and fifth decade. Interestingly, above 60 years of age, all three subtypes had equal distribution.

Subacute presentation was bilateral. Both eyes were affected in 95.5% of subacute PAC, 64.1% of chronic PACG, and only 35.5% of acute PACG. An absolute eye was most often seen with chronic angle-closure glaucoma (32.3%) and following an acute attack (15.3%). About 7% were bilaterally blind. Only 8.9% of the patients who had had an acute PACG achieved a final vision of 20/40 or better. PACG accounts for about half of all glaucoma-related blindness worldwide, despite being less common than open-angle glaucoma globally.

RISK FACTORS

Common risk factors for PACD include:

- *Anatomical factors* which predispose the eye to angle closure include shallow AC depth, small corneal diameter, hyperopia (farsightedness >+3 Diopters), short axial length (<22 mm), and a thick lens (>5 mm), anteriorly positioned crystalline lens, thickened iris or high insertion of iris, and suprachoroidal/ciliary effusion are the nonpupillary block mechanisms contributing to PACD. Increased lens thickness/axial length ratio, increased lens vault >1 mm, and steeper curvature of lens surface anteriorly are other anatomical risk factors predisposing them to angle closure.
- In an interesting study done by Li et al. (2019) in the Chinese population, increase in axial length was found to be associated with severity of PACG in female patients but not in male patients.
- *Asian descent* both East Asians and Indians and also Inuit population
- *Women* are at a higher risk due to shallower ACs and narrower angles
- *Older individuals* are at a higher risk as the lens grows thicker with age, it pushes the iris forward, narrowing the AC further, and closing the angle further.
- *Genetic predisposition* plays a role, and having a family history of PACG increases the risk, especially in the first-degree relatives as anatomic features are inherited.
- Dim lighting causes the pupil to dilate or emotional stress/drugs with a sympathomimetic effect cause a mild dilation of pupil leading to a subacute angle closure in a predisposed eye. Other drugs can also cause angle closure, the list is big, some tricyclic antidepressants, serotonin receptor inhibitors, and some sulfa drugs are known to cause an idiosyncratic reaction leading to supraciliary effusions and angle closure. Some benzodiazepines (BZDs) are γ-aminobutyric acid (GABA) receptor agonists used to treat anxiety, insomnia, and seizure disorders also are

weakly anticholinergic and can affect pupillary sphincter muscle tone and induce pupillary dilation. Topiramate, an antiepileptic medication known to be a risk factor for AACG. Patients with topiramate-induced angle closure present with bilateral involvement and large myopic shifts (up to -17 D). Lens edema and supraciliary effusion induced by topiramate which contribute to forward displacement of the lens-iris diaphragm. Nasal decongestants often contain phenylephrine or pseudoephedrine often paired with antihistamines, which also have anticholinergic effects. The synergistic action of these compounds can dilate the pupil, resulting in a pupillary block. Tamiflu used for influenza is also known to cause an angle closure.

PATHOPHYSIOLOGY

Aqueous humor is produced by the ciliary body, flows through the pupil into the AC, and exits at the AC angle via the trabecular meshwork into Schlemm canal which ultimately drains into the episcleral veins eventually.

The most common physiological mechanism leading to PAC is acknowledged to be a *relative pupillary block*, due to increased iridolenticular contact in anatomically predisposed eyes preventing the free flow of aqueous, produced in the posterior chamber, from passing through the pupil. This increased resistance leads to a pressure differential between the posterior and ACs, causing the peripheral iris to be pushed forward, coming into contact with the intracameral surface of the trabecular meshwork, over a small or large part of its circumferential extent. Ischemic changes are seen more often in the symptomatic patients of angle-closure disease. PACD is more often symptomatic in whites than Asians. Blockage may be appositional or synechial.

Appositional angle closure: Iris rests against and covers the trabecular meshwork; in eyes with a narrow AC angle, dilation increases the iris volume near the periphery, predisposing it to temporary appositional angle closure which may be intermittent.

Synechial angle closure: Iris permanently adheres to trabecular meshwork, owing to fibrosis between the surfaces, this closure does not open up after laser iridotomy. Presence of blotchy pigment in the angle is evidence of angle closure.

Pupillary block: Aqueous humor flows through the pupil but it is obstructed due to relative contact between the iris and lens, pushing the iris forward, leading to closure of AC angle. A blockage of aqueous humor flow from posterior to AC at the pupil; results in increased posterior segment pressure, causing iris to bow anteriorly and narrow or close the angle of the eye. It is the mechanism involved in 75% of cases.

Plateau iris: The peripheral iris is pushed against the trabecular meshwork due to anatomical factors, despite a normal pupillary mechanism. There is an anteriorly positioned ciliary body with deep central AC.

A mid-dilated pupil results in apposition/contact of the anterior lens surface and posterior surface of iris, thus preventing flow of aqueous humor into AC. This pushes the peripheral iris anteriorly blocking the trabecular meshwork, which is reversible and after prolonged contact becomes permanent. The increase in IOP due to this obstruction can damage the ganglion cells of the optic nerve over time producing characteristic changes in the ONH with visual field defects.

Lens-related mechanism (including both the thickness and the anteroposterior position of the crystalline lens), with relative pupil block being the most common mechanism of PACD.

Acute angle-closure glaucoma [also called acute primary angle closure (APAC)] is a medical emergency which occurs in a few cases of PACG. It usually presents unilaterally as a painful sudden loss of vision accompanied with watering, redness, vomiting, nausea, and headache with very high IOP up to 80 mm Hg. It requires immediate lowering of IOP to prevent blindness. Clinically, there is ciliary congestion, fall in vision, with IOP peaking up to 80 mm Hg, corneal edema, shallow AC, vertically oval fixed mid-dilated pupil. In the first attack, the optic disc may be hyperemic without a high cup-disc ratio. Many a time they reach the physician and not an ophthalmologist with severe headache, and may be visual loss, with high IOP and red eye being missed. Pupillary block is the major mechanism contributing to angle closure. The aqueous collected behind the iris pushes the iris diaphragm forward, occluding the AC angle. Iris crowding mechanism and/or anteriorly positioned ciliary body and plateau iris also predispose a patient with narrow angles to AACG. Trigger factors for its occurrence and why it occurs in only a few cases and predictive value of who is more predisposed to it is unknown. Autonomic factors are known to be correlated, sudden swelling of ciliary body—choroidal effusion and ocular inflammation, sympathetic surge as in painful conditions like herpes zoster ophthalmicus causing dilation of pupil and infective states causing AACG have all been reported as contributory factors for AACG and a detailed article by Xhang et al. discusses it well in detail. Inflammatory cytokines are high in aqueous of AACG patients but whether it is the cause, or the result of angle closure has not been ascertained. It is hypothesized that emotional/psychological state also causes choroidal effusion via the autonomic nervous system as it has been seen that psychological states such as depression and anxiety, and post-stress situations like demise of a family member have been known to trigger onset of AACG. A dysfunctional autonomic nervous system may also play a role in triggering AACG. Valsalva's maneuver (forced expiration against a closed airway) causes sudden IOP rise, narrowing of AC angle recess, thickening of the ciliary body which may trigger AACG also. This effect is also produced by blowing wind instruments and conches. AACG has been reported to occur in winter more often in temperate areas, e.g., Finland and during rainy days in the hot tropical areas. We know that anatomic factors like demographic, genetic, psychologic, physiologic, infection, inflammation, and environmental factors all play a role in AACG, but we have not reached a level of understanding to predict and prevent AACG attacks.

SYMPTOMS AND SIGNS

- *History:* Many are asymptomatic or seek an eye consultation for an unrelated complaint, others may have intermittent vision disturbances, pain, headache, or history of glaucoma in the family. Rarely, they may complain of colored haloes or vision loss. Patients of acute angle-closure attack have acute painful visual loss with severe ocular pain, headache, watering, collared haloes, and a red eye.
- *Slit lamp examination:* A shallow AC depth and note the van Herick's (VH) grading. Only VH grade IV peripheral corneal thickness ≥AC depth is free of angle closure. Note the corneal clarity. Iris may show loss of pupillary ruff, sectoral atrophy with abnormal shape of the pupil in the area of atrophy, especially after AACG. A brisk pupillary reaction conveys a healthy optic nerve and a relative afferent pupillary defect conveys severe GON. Lens is thick and anteriorly placed in PACG, a thickness of >5 mm predisposes to AACG. An anterior capsular lenticular opacity (Glaucomflecken-Spilt milk appearance) is seen after angle-closure attack and is a sign of ischemia.
- *Gonioscopy:* Gold standard for visualizing the AC angle and assessing the extent of closure. VH grade I (<1/4 of peripheral corneal thickness), grade II (1/4 of peripheral corneal thickness), and grade III (1/4 to 1/2 peripheral thickness) should all undergo gonioscopy to rule out angle closure. Only VH grade IV and pseudophakes need not undergo gonioscopy to rule out angle closure. All angles where not more than anterior one-third of trabecular meshwork, anterior Schwalbe's line is seen or only dipping of beam is seen in 180° or more are classified as narrow angles.
- *Tonometry:* Applanation tonometry is to be done in every case, an IOP >21 mm Hg is an elevated IOP.
- *Optic nerve evaluation:* It is a must in every case, especially a dilated one (unless contraindicated) as stereoscopic slit lamp biomicroscopy with 90 D lens. Avoid pupil dilation initially, as dilation can precipitate acute angle-closure crisis. A cup-disc ratio of 0.4:1 or more becomes significant in the smaller ONHs found in PACG cases or >0.2 asymmetry between cups, as also notching. Retinal nerve fiber layer and the neuroretinal rim thickness and vascularity need to be assessed. All these findings help to guide treatment goals. It should be drawn or photographed.

- *Optical coherence tomography (OCT):* It is used to assess angle structure and optic nerve. Anterior segment optical coherence tomography (AS-OCT) conveys the angle morphology at only a point. It is not a substitute for gonioscopy which assesses AC angles dynamically. AS-OCT also helps to measure the lens vault.
- *Visual field testing:* To detect visual field loss due to optic nerve damage
- *Anterior segment imaging* is considered when AC angle anatomy is difficult to assess on gonioscopy with *ultrasonographic biomicroscopy (USB)* or *AS-OCT*.
- Some present as an acute attack of angle-closure glaucoma. Acute angle closure is an ocular emergency with symptoms including acute onset of eye pain, blurred vision, headache, nausea, and vomiting. Signs include red eye, fixed and mid-dilated pupil, hazy cornea, and highly elevated IOPs (if >30 mm Hg, needs more than just eyedrops to lower the IOP).

How do you clinch a diagnosis?

Primary angle closure and PACS patients are often asymptomatic, or they may present to you with headache, colored haloes, and blurred vision. Apart from a detailed history of the symptoms, a good history of their systemic diseases and treatment being taken should be obtained.

Very often these patients are hypermetropes. Some may complain of nonspecific symptoms such as a heaviness in the head, mild headache, or very rarely—onset of headache on entering darkly lit places like a cinema hall, and the discomfort subsides after they go back to better lit areas. Dark-room dynamic gonioscopy under topical anesthesia should be performed to diagnose PACD with preferably a four mirror Sussman type of Gonio lens. This should be done in a room with lights switched off using a small 1 mm vertical slit beam less than the size of the pupil in an undilated eye. Angles are narrow if one cannot see beyond the anterior one-third of the trabecular meshwork. In narrow angles, either the beam dips into the angle and none of the structures in the angle can be seen, or the Schwalbe's line is visible. In eyes with narrow angles, 180° or more of the circumference, posterior trabecular meshwork cannot be seen.

In patients with PACS and PACG, IOP may be high; there may be disc and visual field changes. >21 mm Hg IOP is considered as high, although in our Indian population even IOPs of 17 mm Hg is high. Best-corrected visual acuity is normal.

Visual field defects typical of glaucoma are seen in PACG and are more central and show rapid worsening if PACG is untreated.

MANAGEMENT

The principle of treating PACD is to first reverse the anatomical angle closure as far as possible, with the aim of controlling the IOP, in order to prevent glaucomatous progression and blindness.

Management varies based on the stage of the disease. Midperipheral yttrium aluminum garnet (YAG) laser iridotomy is the one procedure that can change the course of the disease. It can be the only curative measure in glaucoma as it opens the angle. It is indicated in all cases PAC and PACG, if the other eye has PAC/PACG, and in PACS if there is a positive family history, one eyed, patients needing repeated dilation for retinal pathology, e.g., diabetics. Use of systemic medications that can provoke pupillary block and angle closure like sympathomimetics/L-dopa, eyes with history suggestive of intermittent angle closure/eyes with progressive narrowing on follow up, patients who cannot come for regular follow-up, and monitoring due to health reasons on geographic location. Unless the patient is on blood thinners, YAG iridotomy can be done anytime. Patient will feel a bit blurred, may have a mild pain, which can be controlled with steroid eyedrops and an IOP rise prevented with a combination of two of these eyedrops brimonidine/ Brinzolamide/dorzolamide and timolol maleate.

Patients of PACS without the abovementioned situations can also be followed annually/biannually to see if they are progressing. They can be counseled about the warning signs of acute attack of angle closure, also to keep pilocarpine 2% available in case they develop symptoms and are unable to reach an eye care facility in time. They also need to be counseled that even after YAG iridotomy, the disease may progress.

Management of AACG: This is a medical emergency requiring immediate attention. We need to give systemic IOP lowering agents:

- *Hyperosmotic agents:* Injection mannitol 1–2 g/kg body weight in three divided doses—for an average 60 kg adult two bottles of 100 cc of 20% mannitol can safely be given. Check blood pressure prior to giving it. Glycerol can also be given orally, but the first choice is mannitol.
- Tablet acetazolamide 250/500 mg stat, repeated 8 hourly till IOP decreases (*Caution:* Avoid it in patients with chronic kidney disease and patients with known allergy to sulfa drugs)
- Timolol (topical β-blockers) and brimonidine (α-agonists) combination can be given twice/thrice daily.
- Prednisolone acetate eyedrops can be given 4 hourly.
- Pilocarpine 2% is effective only when IOP is <40 mm Hg. It can be given three times a day. Prostaglandins can be used as the last resort in uncontrolled IOP.
- Need to recheck IOP and if not getting lowered may need paracentesis to lower it. Once IOP is lowered enough and AC is formed, a YAG laser iridotomy can be attempted. This is the only definitive treatment for acute ACG. Mechanical pressure on the cornea can force the aqueous to be pushed into the angle and help to break an angle closure using a gonioscope.

- Symptomatic treatment for headache, nausea, and vomiting can be given with antiemetics and paracetamol.
- Once the acute phase subsides, IOP comes down and vision may improve. Depending on IOP level, the medications are tapered both for inflammation and elevated pressure. A couple of weeks later, glaucoma evaluation can be done including post-LPI gonioscopy, visual fields, OCT, pachymetry, and fundus photo. The need for long-term antiglaucoma is decided, and patients can be reviewed at 1, 4, and 12 weeks. If the angle closure is synechial and angles do not open in >180° or IOP is uncontrolled despite antiglaucoma medications, trabeculectomy with mitomycin C (MMC) with releasable sutures is indicated to control glaucomatous damage. It may need to be combined with cataract surgery—phacotrabeculectomy in the presence of significant cataract. Cataract surgery alone may be needed for angle closures with a thick lens, high lens vault, or an anteriorly placed intumescent lens.

Initial treatment of acute angle closure is aimed at decreasing IOP. Definitive treatment of angle closure is LPI, with prophylactic iridotomy in the fellow eye, after confirming that it is anatomically narrow. Laser iridoplasty has a limited role in eyes where there is angle crowding with appositional closure, using large size, low intensity, and long duration burns in peripheral iris in order to open the angle. Lens extraction has a limited role in the management of angle closure and can be only reserved for angles that do not open after iridotomy and have a large lens with very shallow AC. Medical treatment for PACG after LPI has a limited role, especially if there is synechial angle closure.

Trabeculectomy is indicated either alone or in combination with cataract surgery—phacoemulsification with a clear corneal incision, when target IOP is not reached even with maximally tolerated medical therapy or glaucoma progression is seen despite IOP control/patient cannot be relied upon taking medical treatment regularly or will be lost to follow up or cannot afford the treatment. An extensive posterior subconjunctival dissection is essential to get diffuse posteriorly directed bleb. Injection MMC 0.01–0.02% sponges/subconjunctival injection is applied for 2–3 minutes to achieve a good functioning bleb that achieves and maintains target IOP over time. 1–2 releasable sutures allow titration of postoperative IOP, and they should be removed only after 1 week, and prevent sudden IOP lowering.

In summary, in India, all eyes that show an anatomical or familial predisposition for *PAC* should have an iridotomy. Patients showing evidence of PAC, i.e., an occludable angle with PAS, with or without a raised IOP, should also have an iridotomy, after controlling any raised IOP. Acute *PACG* eyes present late and frequently require a trabeculectomy to control IOP, but visual prognosis is generally poor. *Chronic PACG* eyes appear to progress faster than POAG eyes. This may be due to continuing periodic angle closure and raised

IOP and due to mechanisms other than relative pupillary block. Antiglaucoma medications should be reevaluated frequently and trabeculectomy may be required if perimetric progression is seen despite topical medication. Trabeculectomy outcomes are good without complications, and success of trabeculectomy is better when antifibrotic medications like MMC are used and releasable sutures are used.

LIVING WITH ANGLE-CLOSURE DISEASE

The prognosis of PACG depends on the stage at which it is diagnosed. PACS and PAC if regularly monitored can preserve vision throughout life. Regular follow-ups should include with eye pressure ONH assessments, visual fields, and OCT. Adherence to medication for IOP is important, also keep in mind the side effects of the topical medications.

Acute angle closure: If treated early, visual outcomes can be favorable. Delays in treatment can lead to permanent optic nerve damage and vision loss.

Chronic angle closure: It often results in gradual visual field loss. Long-term management is aimed at controlling IOP and preventing optic nerve damage. Early diagnosis and intervention are critical in preventing permanent vision loss. Patients should be aware of symptoms such as blurred vision or halos with pain and headache—seek immediate care if an acute attack is suspected.

SCREENING AND PREVENTION

At-risk populations:

- World Glaucoma Association states that angle closure case detection or opportunistic screening should be performed in all persons aged 40 years or older who are undergoing an eye examination. While a shallow AC is strongly associated with angle closure, use of AC depth for population-based screening remains unproven.
- Gonioscopy should be done as a routine in evaluating every glaucoma. Unfortunately, many who treat glaucoma are hesitant in doing gonioscopy neglect it, often omit doing it or perform it inappropriately as evidenced by Chennai Population Study which found that two-thirds of those with PACG were being treated as POAG. Hence, proficiency in performing gonioscopy improves if one does it in every glaucoma suspect with practice, eventually it does not take more than a minute to perform it.
- American Academy of Ophthalmology recommends eye examination for general population, which includes glaucoma screening, by an eye professional for general eye health, for patients with no signs, symptoms, or risk factors for ocular disease: aged 40 years: 1 examination; aged 41–54 years: every 2–4 years; aged 55–64 years: every 1–3 years; and aged 65 years or older: every 1–2 years.

SUGGESTED READING

1. Bhartiya S, Ichhpujani P. Diurnal Intraocular Pressure Fluctuation in Eyes with Angle-closure. J Curr Glaucoma Pract. 2015;9(1):20-3.
2. Li S, Shao M, Wan Y, Tang B, Sun X, Cao W. Relationship between ocular biometry and severity of primary angle-closure glaucoma: relevance for predictive, preventive, and personalized medicine. EPMA J. 2019;10(3):261-71.
3. Sihota R, Angmo D, Ramaswamy D, Dada T. Simplifying "target" intraocular pressure for different stages of primary open-angle glaucoma and primary angle-closure glaucoma. Indian J Ophthalmol. 2018;66(4):495-505.
4. Sihota R, Midha N, Selvan H, Sidhu T, Swamy DR, Sharma A, et al. Prognosis of different glaucomas seen at a tertiary center: A 10-year overview. Indian J Ophthalmol. 2017;65(2):128-32.
5. Sihota R, Shakrawal J, Sharma AK, Gupta A, Dada T, Pandey V. Long-term perimetric stabilization with a management algorithm of set target intraocular pressure in different severities of primary angle-closure glaucoma. Indian J Ophthalmol. 2021:69(10):2721-7.
6. Sihota R. An Indian perspective on primary angle closure and glaucoma. Indian J Ophthalmol. 2011;59 Suppl(Suppl1):S76-81.
7. Sihota R. Classification of primary angle closure disease. Curr Opin Ophthalmol. 2011;22(2):87-95.
8. Sihota R. Classification of primary angle closure disease. Curr Opin Ophthalmol. 2011;22(2):87-95.
9. Wang Y, Guo Y, Zhang Y, Huang S, Zhong Y. Differences and Similarities Between Primary Open Angle Glaucoma and Primary Angle-Closure Glaucoma. Eye Brain. 2024;16:39-54.
10. Zhang X, Liu Y, Wang W, Chen S, Li F, Huang W, et al. Why does acute primary angle closure happen? Potential risk factors for acute primary angle closure. Surv Ophthalmol. 2017;62(5):635-47.

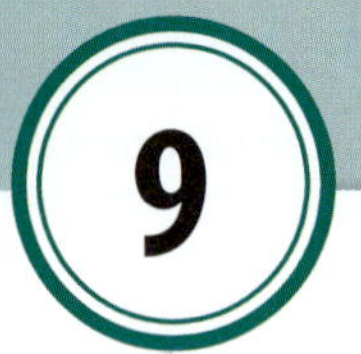

CHAPTER

Primary Open-angle Glaucoma

Rita Dhamankar

INTRODUCTION

A 71-year-old ophthalmologist presented to us with a history of (h/o) diminished vision in BE since around a year. Due to some personal problems, he could not seek help immediately. H/o being diagnosed as ocular hypertension (OHT) around 10 years ago, with highest intraocular pressure (IOP) being recorded as 24 mm Hg in the right eye (RE) and 22 mm Hg in the left eye (LE). And also, he was seen regularly yearly thereafter with no significant changes. In the meanwhile, he was diagnosed to have diabetes, which was well under control a year ago, on medications, with glycated hemoglobin (HbA1c) around 6.5%.

Systemic history: H/o supraventricular tachycardia 15 years ago, undergone an ablation for the same. No h/o hypertension and no h/o any other comorbidities.

Family history: No h/o glaucoma in the family. H/o hypertension in father.

Social history: Nothing specific noted

Allergies: No known drug allergy

Presently on antidiabetic medication

On examination:

- *BCVA 6/24, N12, and 6/9, N8*. No improvement seen with glasses.
- Conjunctiva and cornea were within normal limit (WNL) in BE
- Anterior chamber (AC) was normal in depth and gonioscopy showed wide open angles to the ciliary body band (CBB) in BE.
- Pupil was round, reacting to light briskly.
- Lens in the right eye showed a *nuclear sclerosis (NS) grade 3 with a brown cataract*. LE showed *NS grade 2*.
- IOP was recorded to be *24 mm Hg in the RE and 16 mm Hg in the LE.*
- *Central corneal thickness (CCT)*: 502 and 506 μ

Fundus as shown below **(Figs. 1 and 2)**:

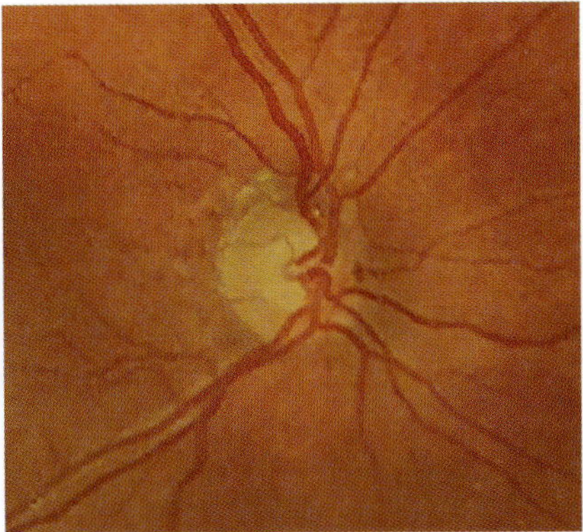

Fig. 1: Right eye fundus.

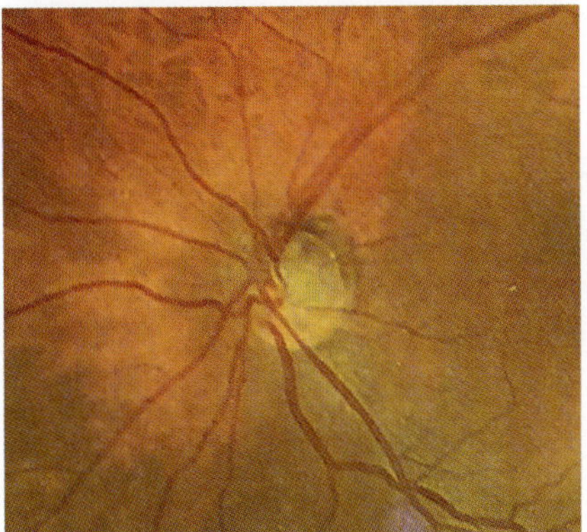

Fig. 2: Left eye fundus.

What will be your provisional diagnosis?

1. Nuclear sclerotic cataracts RE > LE
2. No diabetic retinopathy
3. ?Primary open-angle glaucoma (POAG) BE

What other investigations will you ask for?

You will want to confirm the diagnosis of POAG, right? So, we went ahead and got perimetry and OCT glaucoma done **(Figs. 3 to 5)**.

This is what we found.

Perimetry in the RE definitely shows a superior arcuate defect.

Optical coherence tomography (OCT) shows a thinning of the inferior retinal nerve fiber layer (RNFL) with gross loss of GCC in the RE, with a normal left eye.

So, now you have a definite diagnosis of RE POAG, together with a NS grade 3 cataract in the RE and an early immature senile cataract (IMSC) in the LE.

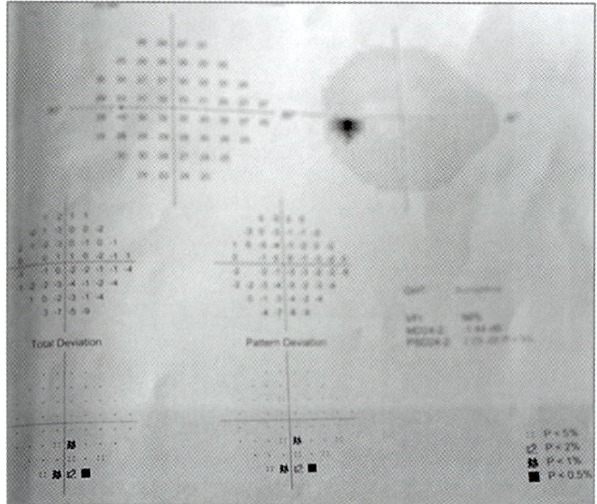

Fig. 3: Left eye 24-2 perimetry.

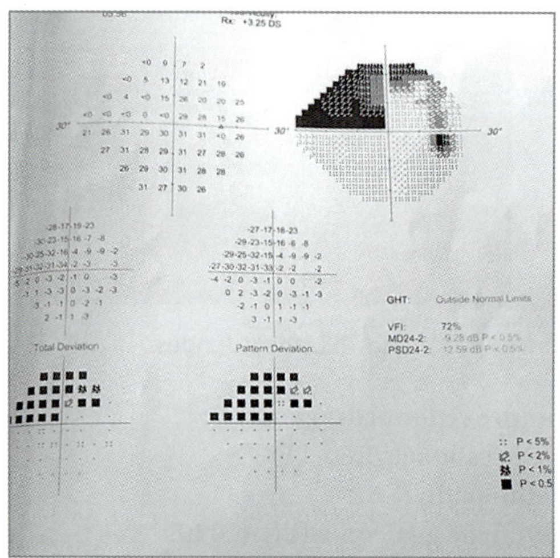

Fig. 4: Right eye 24-2 perimetry.

This entire case was to impress upon you, how silently POAG presents. Here was an ophthalmologist, who was aware of OHT, risk factor of diabetes, getting an eye checkup regularly and yet did not realize how OHT progressed to glaucoma. *90% of patients with POAG* in the underdeveloped world *do not know they have glaucoma*. Here is a glaring example.

Let us move on to see what is POAG all about.

DEFINITION

Primary open-angle glaucoma is a chronic and progressive optic neuropathy in adults wherein, in the presence of an open angle of the anterior chamber,

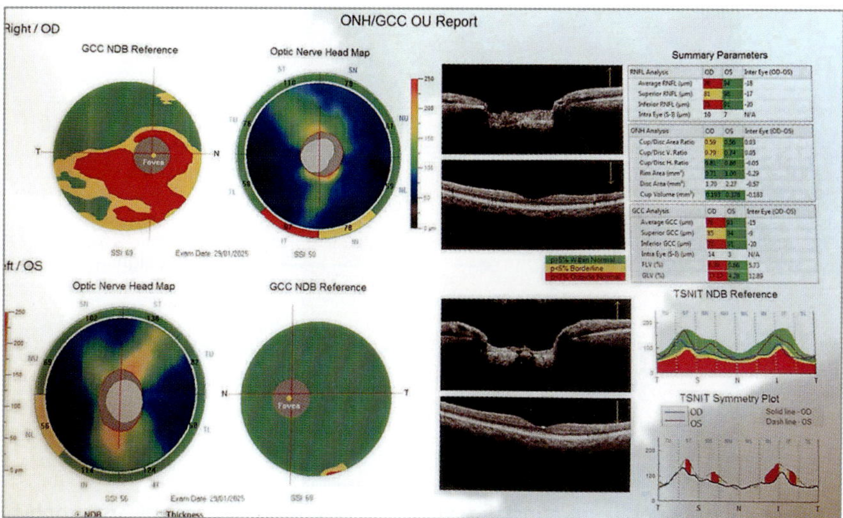

Fig. 5: Optical coherence tomography (OCT) glaucoma both eyes. (GCC: ganglion cell complex; NDB; normative database; ONH: optic nerve head)

there is a characteristic acquired atrophy of the optic nerve and loss of retinal ganglion cells and their axons without any other contributing pathology.

INCIDENCE OF PRIMARY OPEN-ANGLE GLAUCOMA

In 2020, approximately 53 million individuals worldwide were diagnosed with POAG, showing a prevalence rate of 3.0% among individuals aged 40–80 years. It is estimated that by 2040, 111.8 million individuals will be living with glaucoma globally, the lion's share of which will be in Asia and Africa. This is of particular concern for us in Asia. Over 5 years, several studies have shown the incidence of new onset of glaucomatous damage in previously unaffected patients to be about 2.6–3% for IOPs 21–25 mm Hg, 12–26% incidence for IOPs 26–30 mm Hg, and approximately 42% for those higher than 30 mm Hg. Hence, we can conclude that though high IOP does not equate to glaucoma, it is certainly a very important risk factor.

SIGNS

Structural changes in the optic disc or retinal nerve fiber which can be identified as:

- Diffuse or focal narrowing, or notching, of the optic disc rim, especially at the inferior or superior poles
- Progressive narrowing of the neuroretinal rim (NRR) with an associated increase in cupping of the optic disc
- Diffuse or localized abnormalities of the parapapillary RNFL, especially at the inferior or superior poles

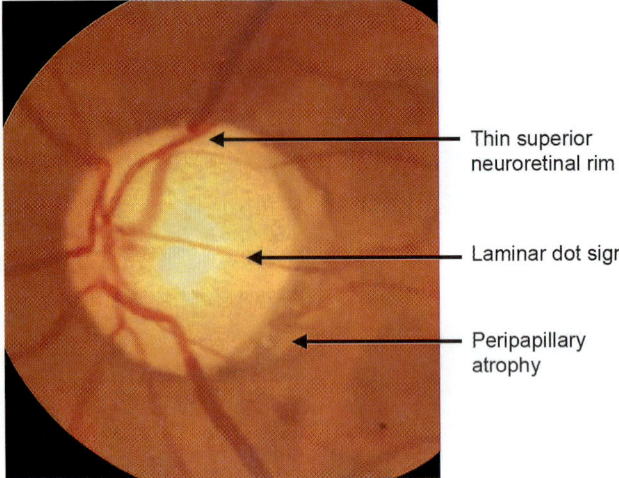

Fig. 6: Thin superior neuroretinal rim, a laminar dot sign and a peripapillary atrophy.

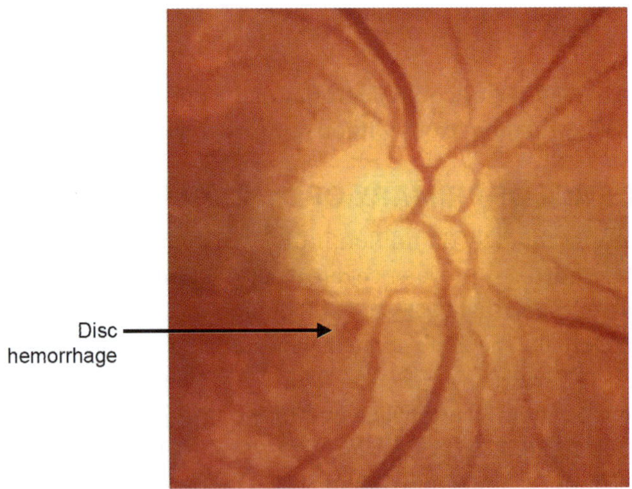

Fig. 7: Sign of progression of Glaucoma.

- Disc rim, parapapillary RNFL, or lamina cribrosa hemorrhages
- Optic disc neural rim asymmetry of the two eyes consistent with loss of neural tissue wherein the difference in the cup-disc ratio is >0.2.
- May be associated with a large extent of parapapillary atrophy **(Fig. 6)**.

Increased cupping, thin NRR, nasalization of vessels, and disc hemorrhage laminar dot sign peripapillary atrophy ***(Fig. 7)***.

Functional changes in the form of reliable and reproducible visual field defects representing the above structural defects **(Fig. 8)**:

- Visual field damage consistent with RNFL damage (e.g., nasal step, arcuate field defect, or paracentral depression in clusters of test sites)

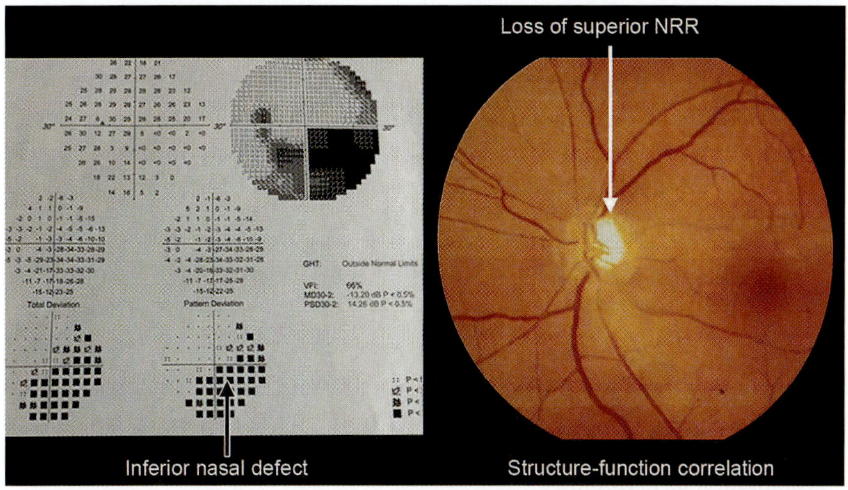

Fig. 8: Inferior nasal defect. Structure-function correlation (NRR: neuroretinal rim)

- Visual field loss across the horizontal midline in one hemifield that exceeds loss in the opposite hemifield (in early/moderate cases)
- Absence of other known explanations (e.g., optic disc drusen and optic nerve pit)

Absence of other known explanations (i.e., secondary glaucoma) for the progressive glaucomatous optic nerve change [e.g., pigment dispersion, pseudoexfoliation (PEX) (exfoliation syndrome), uveitis, trauma, and corticosteroid use].

Primary open-angle glaucoma represents a *spectrum of disease in adults* in which the susceptibility of the optic nerve to damage varies among patients. Most patients with *POAG present with raised IOP*, however, almost *40%* of those with the abovementioned characteristic changes in the disc *may have IOP within the normal range*. These are classified as *normal tension glaucoma (NTG).*

There is also another spectrum of patients who may present with an elevated IOP, but with no changes in the optic nerve head, these are labeled as *OHT*.

Depending on the severity of damage, POAG is classified as mild, moderate, and severe:

- *Mild:* Definite optic disc or RNFL abnormalities consistent with glaucoma as detailed above and a normal visual field as tested with standard automated perimetry (SAP)
- *Moderate:* Definite optic disc or RNFL abnormalities consistent with glaucoma as detailed above and visual field abnormalities in one hemifield that are not within 5° of fixation as tested with SAP.

- *Severe:* Definite optic disc or RNFL abnormalities consistent with glaucoma as detailed above and visual field abnormalities in both hemifields and/or loss within 5° of fixation in at least one hemifield as tested with SAP
- *Indeterminate:* Definite optic disc or RNFL abnormalities consistent with glaucoma as detailed above, inability of patient to perform visual field testing, unreliable/uninterpretable visual field test results, or visual fields not performed yet

What is the clinical perspective after making a diagnosis of POAG?
Knowing that *progression of POAG* can lead to *irreversible blindness.*

We need to:

- Document the status of optic nerve structure and function on presentation
- Estimate an IOP below which further optic nerve damage is unlikely to occur (target IOP) as reduction of IOP is the only known treatment for glaucoma as of today.
- Try and maintain this range of IOP by appropriate medical/laser and/or surgical intervention(s).
- Continue monitoring the structure and function of the optic nerve for progression and adjust the target IOP accordingly.
- Try to keep the side effects of treatment and their impact on the patient's vision, general health, to a minimum. Thus, ensuring a good quality of life.
- Spend adequate chair time, educating both the patient and the caregivers about the disease, and the need for compliance of treatment and regular monitoring.

Who is at a risk?

- Higher IOP
- Older age
- Family history of glaucoma
- African race or Latino/Hispanic ethnicity
- Patients with a history of ocular trauma/surgery
- Type 2 diabetes mellitus
- Myopia
- Lower systolic and diastolic blood pressure
- Patients on long-term steroids
- Other factors—migraine, vasospasm, systemic arterial hypertension, cerebrospinal fluid pressure, and genetic factors

ROLE OF INTRAOCULAR PRESSURE

Though IOP finds no place in the definition of glaucoma, many studies have shown that the prevalence of POAG increases with a rise in the IOP. Also, studies have proven that decreasing the IOP by any means is the only treatable parameter in glaucoma.

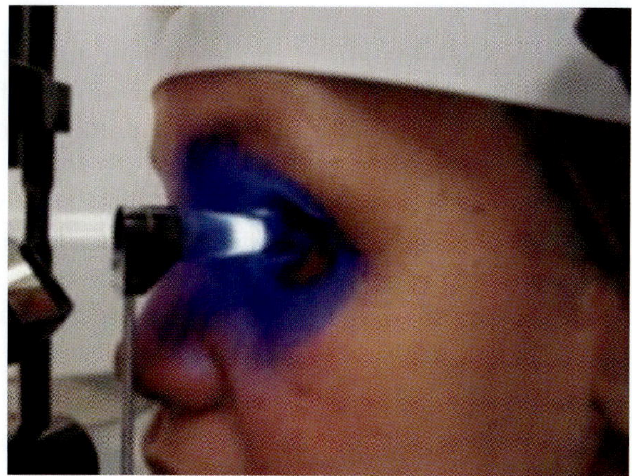

Fig. 9: Goldmann applanation tonometry (GAT).
Source: Richard Scawn. Applanation tonometry, UK.

Hence, though IOP is not the identifying parameter, it plays a very important role in the management of glaucoma and needs to be measured at every visit.

How is IOP measured?

The gold standard of measuring the IOP is the Goldmann applanation tonometer (GAT) **(Fig. 9)**.

In a busy outpatient department (OPD), however the noncontact tonometry is very useful for *screening.*

What is the best way to identify glaucoma in society, as this is a major health problem, leading to irreversible blindness? Can we resort to screening in the population at large? The answer is *NO.*

Whom do we screen?

As the disease is a *silent thief of sight,* most patients do not seek help till the disease is very advanced, hence, diagnosing glaucoma early and starting treatment definitely helps in preventing blindness.

Whom do you screen, if not the entire population? We have had a look at all the risk factors. All patients above the age of 40 years, with a family history of glaucoma, may be myopes, diabetic, have a h/o ocular trauma/surgery, and may be the target population that can be screened and give very good results.

What all needs to be looked at?

There are three main approaches to screening patients for POAG: *(1) measuring the IOP, (2) assessing the ONH and RNFL, and (3) evaluating the visual field, either alone or in combination.* Measuring IOP alone is not an effective method for screening populations for glaucoma.

How does one proceed?

A comprehensive eye examination of the eye including a gonioscopy, measurement of the IOP, evaluation of the disc structurally, and functionally is a must, after the detailed initial history is taken to come to a diagnosis of glaucoma.

The aim is to make a correct diagnosis. Set a target IOP and try to achieve it by initiating therapy as is deemed most effective and least toxic, yet being affordable, so as to prevent progression of the disease. This does not happen in one visit. Repeat follow-ups, monitoring the disc, the fields and the IOP over the lifetime helps you get there.

Start with a detailed history including:

- *Ocular history* (e.g., refractive error, trauma, and prior ocular surgery)
- Race/ethnicity
- *Family history:* The severity and outcome of glaucoma in family members, including a history of visual loss from glaucoma, should be obtained during initial evaluation.
- Systemic history, e.g., asthma/chronic obstructive pulmonary disease, migraine headache, vasospasm, diabetes, and cardiovascular disease
- Review of pertinent records with particular reference to the past IOP levels, status of the optic nerve, and visual field
- Current ocular, topical, oral, injected, or inhaled medications (e.g., corticosteroids) and known local or systemic intolerance to ocular or nonocular medications

Ocular surgery: A history of LASIK or photorefractive keratectomy is associated with a falsely low IOP measurement due to thinning of the cornea. Cataract surgery may also lower the IOP compared with the presurgical baseline. A history of prior glaucoma laser or incisional surgical procedures should be elicited.

The comprehensive eye examination includes:

- *Visual acuity* measurement for distance and near
- *Pupil examination:* Look for pupillary abnormalities and reaction.
- *Anterior segment examination* includes examination of all the anterior segments including the anterior chamber, iris, and lens
- *Gonioscopy:* To look for all the visible structures in the angle, after assessing it is open.
- *IOP* measurement on the GAT
- *ONH and RNFL with a stereofundus examination:* The fundus examination should be done with a dilated pupil with a condensing lens on a slit lamp, to ensure all the details are picked up which includes a search for other abnormalities that may account for optic nerve changes and/or visual field defects (e.g., disc drusen, optic nerve pits, disc edema or pallor from central nervous system disease or anterior ischemic optic neuropathy,

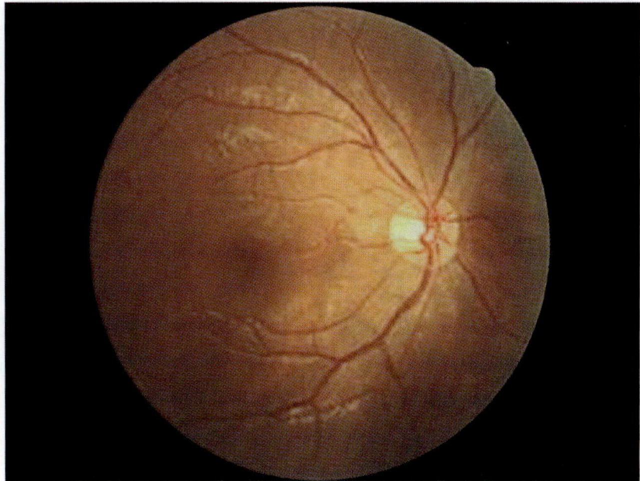

Fig. 10: Normal fundus.

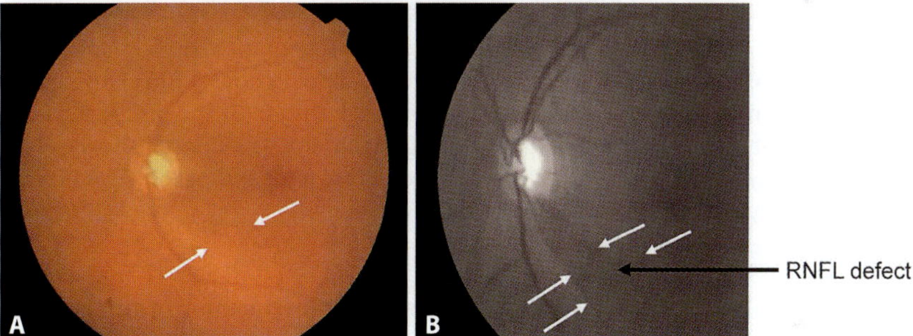

Figs. 11A and B: (A) Normal image of the fundus RNFL defect; (B) Red free filter so the RNFL shows up like a dark defect.

macular degeneration, retinovascular occlusion, or other retinal disease) **(Figs. 10 and 11)**.

What do you look for?

- Look for vertical elongation of the optic cup with associated decrease in neuroretinal rim width
- Excavation of the cup
- Thinning of the RNFL
- Notching and/or thinning of the neuroretinal rim
- Disc hemorrhage!
- Large extent of parapapillary atrophy
- Nasalization of central ONH vessels
- Baring of the circumlinear vessel
- Absence of neuroretinal rim pallor

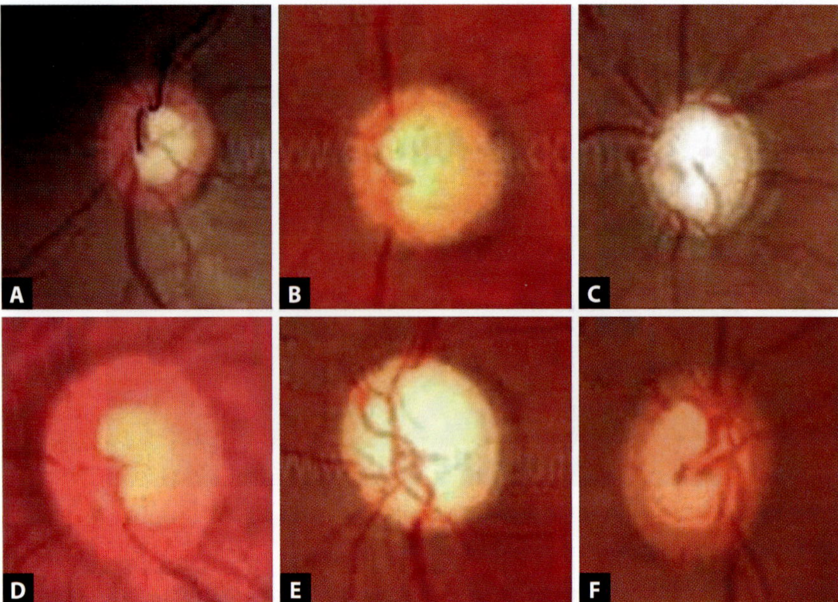

Figs. 12A to F: Different disc pictures showing a variety of glaucoma changes. (A) Bayoneting sign, at 12 o'clock you can see the vessel dipping down; (B) Enlarged cup-disc ratio, with nasalization of vessels and a laminar dot sign; (C) The disc is showing an optic disc pit at 9 o'clock; (D) Disc suspect; (E) Again the superior rim shows a less well-defined bayoneting sign with a very large cup-disc (c/d) and pallor; (F) A bipolar thinning, slightly tilted disc, with nasalization of vessels.

The normal NRR follows the ISNT pattern wherein the inferior rim is wider than the superior rim which is thicker than the nasal rim which is thicker than the temporal rim, i.e., I>S>N>T. Any change in this configuration should be looked at with caution **(Figs. 12A to F)**.

- Look at the entire retina to search for other retinal problems that can mimic visual field changes as mentioned above.

Having made a diagnosis of a glaucomatous disc, we proceed to doing a few mandatory tests:

- Perimetry to look at visual field defects look in the chapter on Perimetry for details. The pearl to be remembered is *always correlate all your perimetry findings with your fundus findings*. This is very important, for an age-related macular degeneration (ARMD) could give you a central defect, which could change your classification of glaucoma, or a branch vein occlusion can show up as an arcuate defect and mimic a glaucoma visual field defect.
- Imaging or optical coherence tomography to look at the structural defects in terms of RNFL defects and ganglion cell complex (GCC) loss. Look in the chapter on imaging for details.

- Try and match your structural defects with the visual field changes too and *a good structure function correlation strengthens your diagnosis.*
- *Central corneal thickness using a pachymeter/anterior segment optical coherence tomography (AS-OCT):* This is an important parameter, as the IOP that is measured through the GAT is calibrated, considering the CCT to be 520 µm. If the cornea is thinner than that, the reading you get will be lesser than what the IOP actually is and vice versa, a thicker cornea yields a false higher reading. There is no standardized algorithm/correction factor and hence, you cannot make a mathematical conversion. However, it is important to remember that *thinner corneas are known to progress faster,* so when setting a target IOP that is something to be thought of. Remember you have to be *aggressive when treating patients with thin corneas.*
- At the end of this you should be fairly confident about making a diagnosis of glaucoma. *A word of Caution.* There exist a lot of glaucoma masquerades. You have to be aware of those, so you do not go astray.

Optic Disc Abnormalities

- Anterior ischemic optic neuropathies
- Optic nerve drusen
- Myopic tilted optic nerves
- Toxic optic neuropathies
- Congenital pit
- Congenital disc anomalies (e.g., coloboma, periventricular leukomalacia, and morning glory syndrome)
- Leber hereditary optic neuropathy and dominant optic atrophy
- Optic neuritis

Retinal Abnormalities

- Age-related macular degeneration
- Panretinal photocoagulation
- Retinitis pigmentosa
- Retinal arterial and venous occlusions

Central Nervous System Abnormalities

- Compressive optic neuropathy
- Demyelination from multiple sclerosis
- Nutritional optic neuropathy
- Dominant optic atrophy

MANAGEMENT

The goal of management of glaucoma is to maintain the target IOP, so as to prevent progression, i.e., a stable visual field.

This can be achieved by medications, laser, or surgery.

The ideal treatment should be maximally effective with minimal side effects and affordable. It should also maintain a good quality of life.

Laser: Selective Laser Trabeculoplasty

It is a Q-switched frequency doubled Nd-YAG laser 532 nM, which targets the pigmented cells without disturbing the nonpigmented cells, with a pulse of 3 ns and a spot size of 400 μm. After instilling a topical anesthetic agent using a Latina gonio lens, you identify the pigmented trabecular meshwork (TM). Aim the Laser beam on the pigmented TM and using an energy of around 8 mJ, start delivering the laser shot till you can just see a bubble. That is the end point. Lower the energy slightly and continue with the laser shots alongside one another so as to cover the entire pigmented TM placing 50 shots in 3 clock hours. The mechanism of the selective laser trabeculoplasty (SLT) is said to be threefold **(Figs. 13 and 14)**.

1. *Cellular:* It suggests that the reduction in IOP occurs due to the cellular activity stimulated by the laser; there is increased recruitment of macrophages in the TM, which aids in the remodeling of the extracellular matrix, thus allowing for increased aqueous outflow.
2. *Cytokine production:* There is increased expression and secretion of Interleukin-1β (IL-1β) and tumor necrosis factor-α (TNF-α) in the first 8 hours after treatment; these mediate increased trabecular stromelysin expression, which leads to remodeling of the juxtacanalicular extracellular matrix of the TM. This improves the normal outflow facility, thereby decreasing IOP.

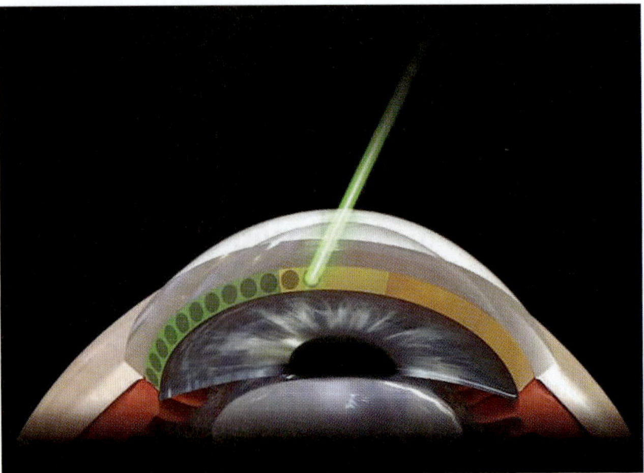

Fig. 13: Application of selective laser trabeculoplasty (SLT) to the pigmented trabecular meshwork. Spot size is large.

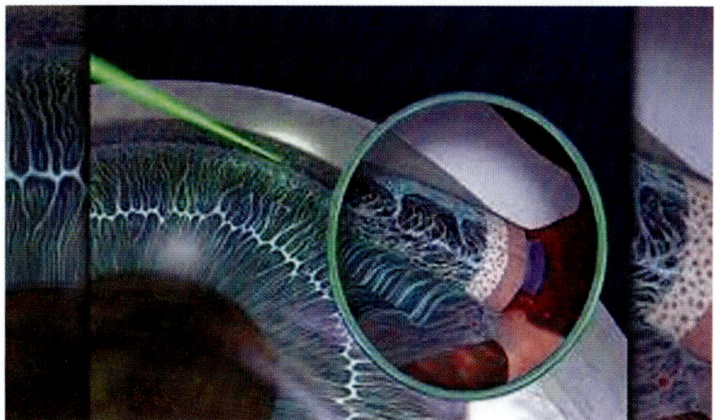

Fig. 14: Identifying the pigmented trabecular meshwork to focus the laser on the pigmented cells.

3. *The increased conductivity* of Schlemm's canal—SLT leads to a threefold increase in Schlemm's canal cells conductivity, thus increasing the transendothelial fluid flow across Schlemm's canal cells.
4. *SLT:* It causes *cracking of intracytoplasmic pigment granules* and disruption of the endothelial cells of the TM.

   This leads to an increase in the outflow mechanism and reduction of IOP.

Complications of SLT

- *Spike in IOP and low-grade iritis:* The spike in IOP can be prevented by using an α-agonist, preprocedure, which can also cause miosis on instillation and helps open the angle wider for better exposure of the angle.
- It may lead to corneal edema, in case of reactivation of an old herpetic infection.

The IOP is known to keep getting lower for a considerable time after the procedure. SLT acts best in a treatment naïve eye, giving up to 30% reduction in IOP. SLT maintains a flat diurnal curve. The effect lasts from 6 months to 5 years. There is a lot of individual variation. However, SLT is repeatable. SLT prevents exposure to toxic preservatives and preserves the health of the conjunctiva. It is very useful in PEX glaucoma, pigmentary glaucoma, and in noncompliant patients. In pregnancy with POAG, and when surgery needs to be deferred for some reason.

Contraindications

- Angle-closure glaucoma
- Inflammatory glaucoma
- Advanced glaucoma

Safety profile: SLT is safe and has a good safety profile. It is associated with fewer adverse events than eye drops.

- *Effectiveness:* SLT is as effective as topical medications. In the Laser in Glaucoma and Ocular Hypertension (LiGHT) trial, SLT achieved drop-free disease control in about 75% of eyes at 3 years.
- *Cost:* SLT is cost-effective compared to medications and more invasive surgeries.
- *Quality of life:* SLT can improve quality of life and reduce the number of topical complications.
- *Repeatability:* SLT can be repeated effectively without damaging the TM.

The *LIGHT trial* has proven that SLT should replace medical management as first line of treatment in POAG as 75% of patients with SLT remained drop free at the end of 3 years, with a better quality of life.

Medical Management of Glaucoma (Fig. 15)

As we have learnt from so many randomized clinical trials (RCTs) that the only known parameter that can dampen/slow the progression in all glaucoma is reduction of the IOP. While we discussed the laser in POAG earlier, let us now move on to the medical management of glaucoma. In the introduction, I have dealt with the concept of target IOP. So, let us revisit it. We know that reduction in IOP works, but how much do we reduce the IOP to? Is there a known algorithm used universally? Well yes or no because the concept of target IOP is to get to an IOP where there will be no progression and how do we estimate that in the clinic for an individual patient? Many consensus reports have now concluded that there are multiple parameters to look at **(Fig. 16)**.

- Age of the patient at presentation
- Damage seen on the disc and fields
- IOP on presentation

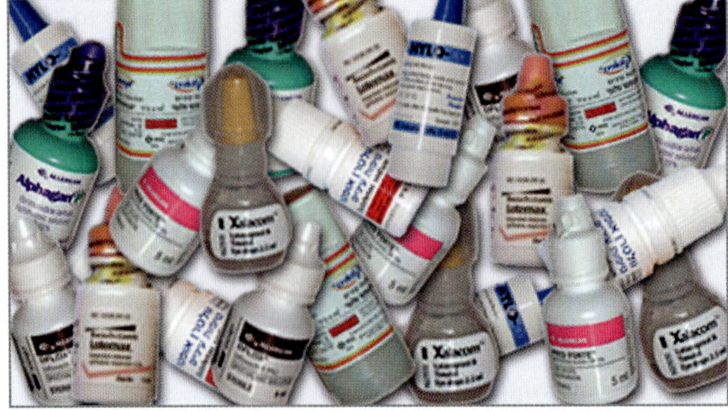

Fig. 15: Look at the number of medications that are available to us for treating glaucoma.

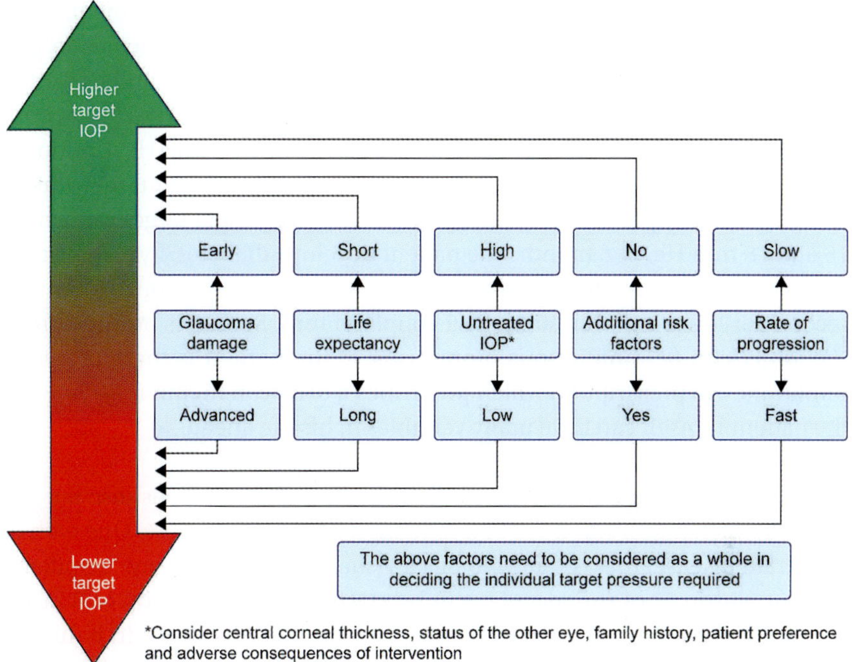

Fig. 16: EGS guidelines on how to calculate the target IOP. (EGS: European Glaucoma Society; IOP: intraocular pressure)
Source: European Glaucoma Society.

- Risk factors such as thin corneas and disc hemorrhages
- Rate of progression

Obviously, you have to be more aggressive in a young patient as he has many more years to live on with the disease, as compared to a relatively older person, say past 75 years, where the chances of him going blind in the next few years of his life are few.

If the disease is diagnosed relatively early, you can be less aggressive as compared to advanced disease.

If the IOP on presentation is high, the lowering has to be more, whereas if the IOP is in the early 20s you may be a little lax and bring it down to may be high teens.

The presence of risk factors will increase the chances of progression, hence, the target IOP should be lower in those patients compared to those with no known risk factors. Obviously, a rapid progressor needs to have very low pressures, sometimes down to the episcleral venous pressures, and those with a slow rate of progression, can continue to stay on a relatively higher target pressure.

The important thing about the *target pressure* is that it is a *range* and not a fixed number and that it is *dynamic*. For example, when you say you would target a patient to be in the high teens it could vary between 16 and

18 mm Hg and not 16 or 18 mm Hg. Similarly, when you start treatment, your guesstimate was high teens and the patient needs three molecules to get there, but over a year, you see, the patient is absolutely stable and finds the treatment to be either complex or he has a lot of side effects of the drugs, you may lessen a drug and raise the target between 18 and 20 mm Hg. Continue monitoring him and if he continues to be stable, the changed target which is higher than originally set is fine. Sometimes, your initial target was set at 16 and 18 mm Hg, in 6 months the patient develops diabetes/hypertension/ needs to be put on steroids for a new systemic disease, you might want to reconsider lowering your target by a couple of mm. So that is how *dynamic the target can be*. Continuous monitoring of the patient is therefore very important. No prescription which prescribes a drug can mention *lifelong*, as the patient himself can have many variables in his life ahead.

There is another simple way of getting to the target.

A patient with a mild disease, which shows a glaucomatous disc but no visual field changes, can do with a reduction of his IOP by 20%. One with a moderate disease, that is one who has a visual field defect in one hemifield but not within 5° of the macula, can be stable with a reduction of 30% of the IOP. One with an advanced disease, i.e., visual field defects in both the hemifields or one hemifield and a paracentral defect within 5° from the macula will need a much lower IOP could go <40–50% of the baseline IOP or even to the episcleral pressures. However, we also have findings from the Advanced Glaucoma Intervention Study (AGIS) which concludes that having an average IOP ≤18 mm Hg at all times is proven to prevent progression **(Tables 1 and 2)**.

TABLE 1: Setting target IOP—numbers or percentages?

Stage of glaucoma	*Evidence*	*IOP percentage reduction*	*Range of IOP*	*Findings from study*
OHTN	OHTS	≥20%	18–21 mm Hg	5% progression at 20% reduction
Mild glaucoma	EMGT, CIGTS	≥25%	<18 mm Hg	30% reduction → no progression in 7 years
Moderate glaucoma	CIGTS, AGIS	≥30%	14–16 mm Hg	
Severe glaucoma	AGIS	≥35%	10–12 mm Hg	IOP average = 12; no progression × 14 years

(AGIS: Advanced Glaucoma Intervention Study; CIGTS: Collaborative Initial Glaucoma Treatment Study; EMGT: Early Manifest Glaucoma Trial; IOP: intraocular pressure; OHTN: ocular hypertension; OHTS: Ocular Hypertension Treatment Study)

TABLE 2: AAO guidelines on getting to the target IOP.

Clinical conditions	*Target IOP*
Glaucoma patients with mild damage (optic disc cupping but no VF loss)	Reduction of 20–30% from baseline
Glaucoma patients with advance damage	Reduction of 40% or more from baseline
Normal pressure glaucoma or NTG	Reduction of 30% from baseline
Ocular hypertension	Reduction of 20% from baseline
Open-angle glaucoma with IOP in the mid to high 20s	Target IOP range 14–18 mm Hg
Advanced glaucoma	Target IOP <15 mm Hg
OHT whose IOP >30 mm Hg with no sign of optic nerve damage	Target IOP <20 mm Hg

(AAO: American Academy of Ophthalmology; IOP: intraocular pressure; NTG: normal-tension glaucoma; OHT: ocular hypertension; VF: visual field)

AAO Guidelines: Target IOP

Having decided on the target, you must decide what are the medications available to you?

The *ideal drug* is one that gives you maximal efficacy, with minimum toxicity, lease dosage, and is affordable, also helps to maintain a good quality of life.

Today, we have many molecules available to us and if we look at the history of medications available, we have as many drugs and as many combinations as you can dream of. You can give 1–3 molecules in one drop. So, you can actually give five molecules in two drops. The question is do so many drops add up mathematically to give you as much reduction. If molecule A gives you a 30% reduction, molecule B gives you a 20% reduction, and molecule C gives you an 18% reduction, remember combining A + B + C will not give you 68% reduction. Once the first molecule has been maximally efficacious, the second will neither give its optimal reduction nor the third one can add much more. Therefore, just adding molecule after molecule is useless. Also, there are some molecules which help production of aqueous and others help aqueous outflow. Adding two outflow facilitators or two aqueous suppressants will never be beneficial. Instead, if the drugs have different modes of action, you are likely to get better results. Remember the second drug must give you at least a 15% reduction after the maximal effect of the first drug. Or else, you are only adding more side effects and are not helping the pressure come down anymore. A detailed chapter on medical management is added to the book, so I will only add special tips in medical management **(Flowcharts 1 and 2 and Figs. 17 and 18)**.

Flowchart 1: Algorithm for medical management of glaucoma.

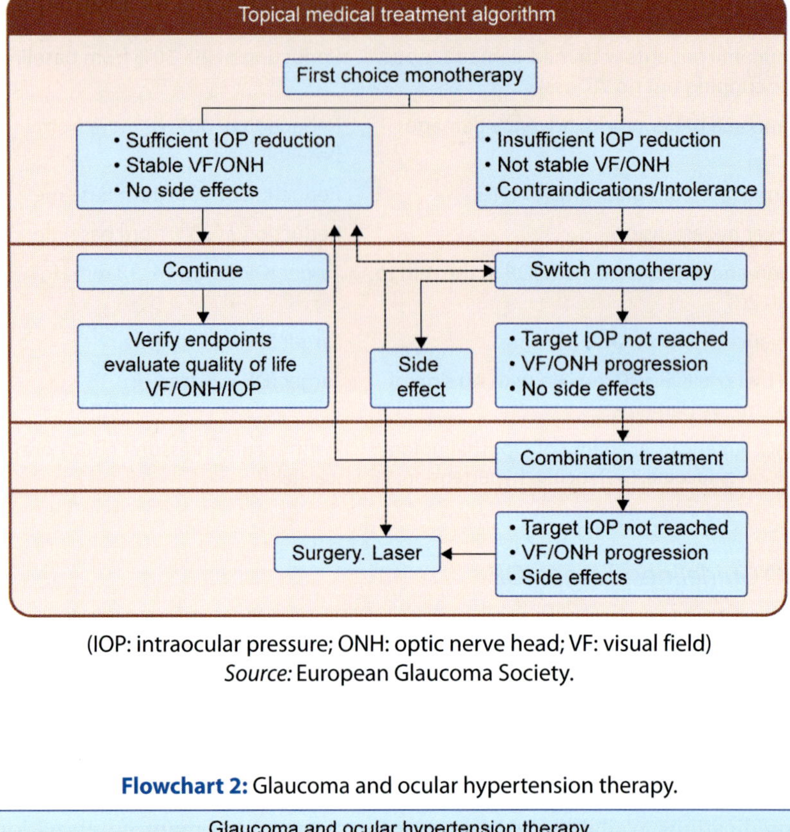

(IOP: intraocular pressure; ONH: optic nerve head; VF: visual field)
Source: European Glaucoma Society.

Flowchart 2: Glaucoma and ocular hypertension therapy.

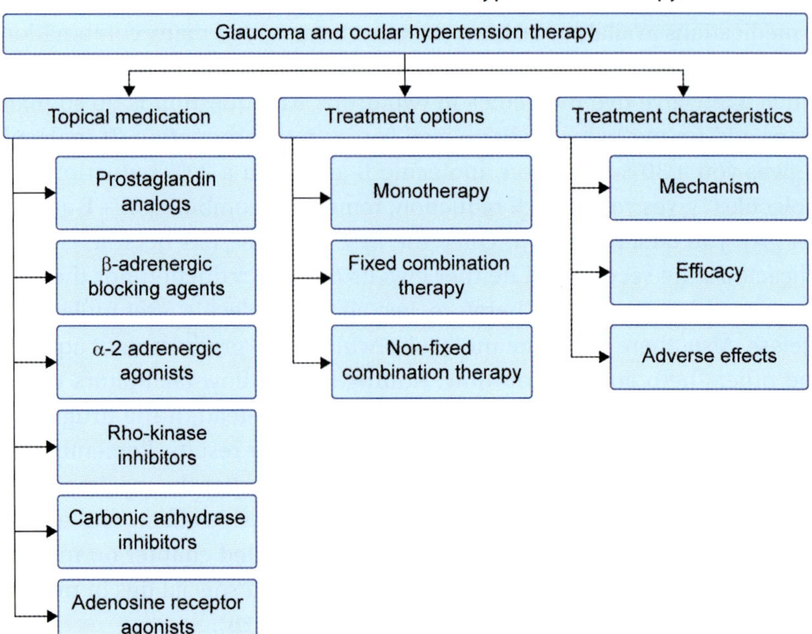

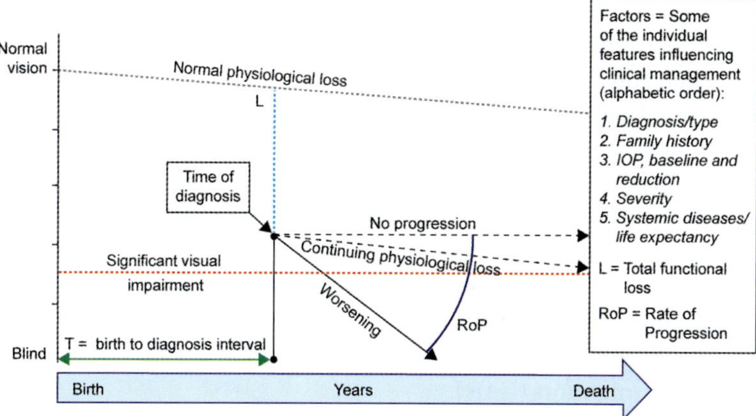

Fig. 17: Graphical representation of the rate of progression in glaucoma. Factors responsible, what treatment can do? When is significant visual impairment noticed? (IOP: intraocular pressure)
Source: European Glaucoma Society.

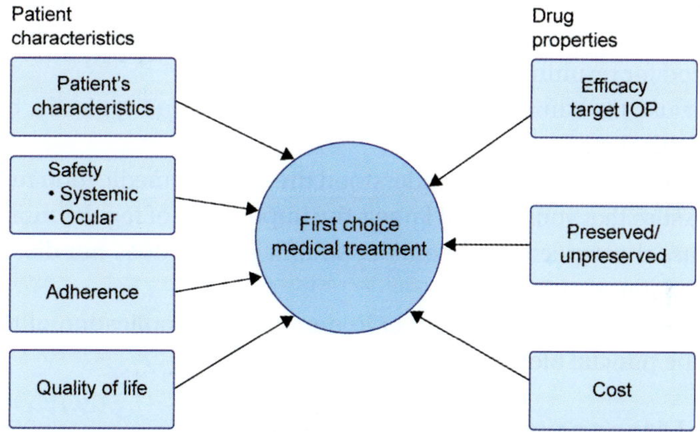

Fig. 18: What influences the physician when making a choice of medical treatment (IOP: intraocular pressure)
Source: European Glaucoma Society.

Pearls of medical management:

- Always estimate the target IOP
- Try to get there with a drug that gets you there
- Make sure the dosing is simple.
- When adding the next drug, ensure it has a different mechanism of action.
- Do not go on adding one medication after another, as the sum effect of the medications is not a mathematical addition.

- When you start medication, always start with a single drug, so you know its efficacy and its tolerability too.
- If needed add a second drug
- If the two drugs are available in a combination therapy, you may opt for a combination therapy, as the exposure to preservatives is reduced, so also the number of drops instilled. This definitely improves compliance.
- If you need to get a large drop in IOP, a systemic medication like acetazolamide is very useful.
- Remember to use potassium supplements with acetazolamide. Never use it in patients allergic to sulfas.
- Patients with a compromised cornea should never be given carbonic anhydrase inhibitors (CAIs).
- Never use prostaglandins in the presence of an inflammation or in case of a compromised posterior capsule.
- Always add medications in a stepwise fashion
- Look for both the efficacy and side effects. Most importantly, look for compliance. Drugs act only when they are used.
- Always ensure that the drugs prescribed are affordable for the patient
- Never prescribe a complicated drug regimen to the patient, it is a sure method for resulting in noncompliance.
- Never use the same molecule both systemically and topically, e.g., CAI and β-blocker.
- Make sure the patient has understood the need for medication regularly.
- Make sure that your patient knows the importance of regular monitoring
- Discuss the expected side effects, so that patient does not discontinue medications on his own.
- At the end, please do not forget to demonstrate application of the drop and the punctal block.

Medical Management in Special Situations

Pregnancy and Breastfeeding

Medical management of glaucoma presents many challenges in pregnancy and breastfeeding mothers, as you want to restrict progression of the disease in the mother and have no effects on the fetus/breastfeeding infant.

Drugs like *prostaglandins* may induce uterine contraction and induce preterm labor and are best avoided in last trimester of pregnancy. β-blockers and carbonic acid inhibitors seem to be relatively safe and may be used both during pregnancy and lactation, though the breastfeeding infant needs to be monitored. *Brimonidine* is a *NO* in infants till the age of 8 years, as it is known to cause respiratory depression. In breastfeeding infants too, it crosses the blood–brain barrier and should *not* be used.

Brimonidine is known to *induce drowsiness* in patients and must be avoided in patients who need to be alert at all times, e.g., drivers and pilots.

Surgical Management of Glaucoma

A special chapter dedicated to surgical management of glaucoma has been described elsewhere; so, here I will just make a mention of the highlights of the surgical treatment.

Incisional surgical treatment for glaucoma, wherein a different pathway for the pooled aqueous is made which is an effective way to prevent progression of glaucoma. The time-tested surgery which has proven to be the gold standard surgery is *trabeculectomy* **(Fig. 19)**.

Trabeculectomy may be resorted to, if the patient continues to progress despite laser, medical management being tried earlier. Sometimes, it may be offered as the first line of therapy in patients presenting with a very advanced disease.

Estimates of success rates over time range from 31 to 88% in different populations and with varying definitions of success and failure. The failure rate of trabeculectomy, without the use of adjunctive antifibrotic medications alone or combined with medical therapy, in a previously unoperated eye in the AGIS reached approximately 30% in African American patients and 20% in Caucasian American patients over a 10-year period.

The use of intraoperative antifibrotic agents has increased the success of trabeculectomy over the years **(Figs. 20 and 21)**.

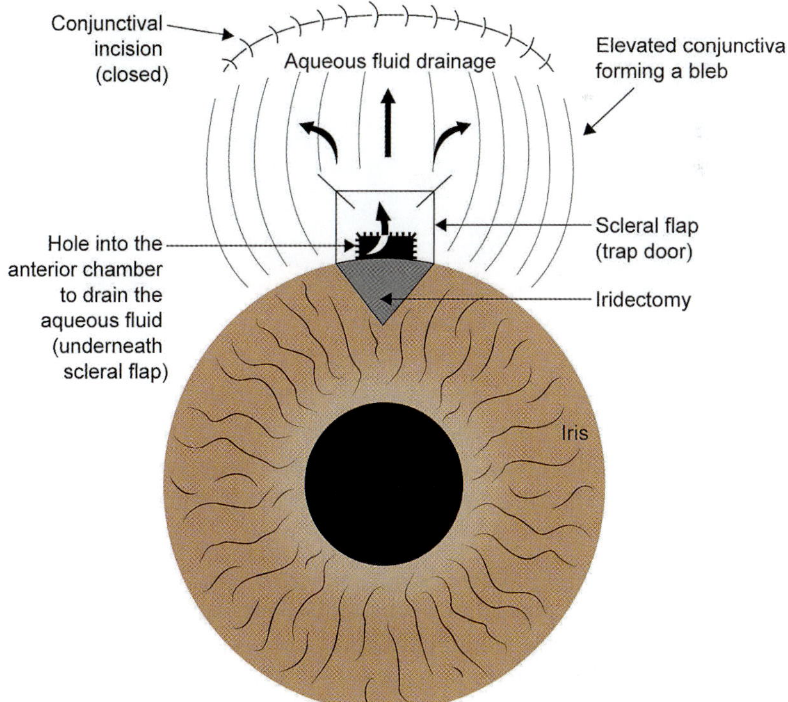

Fig. 19: Trabeculectomy with a limbal-based conjunctival flap.

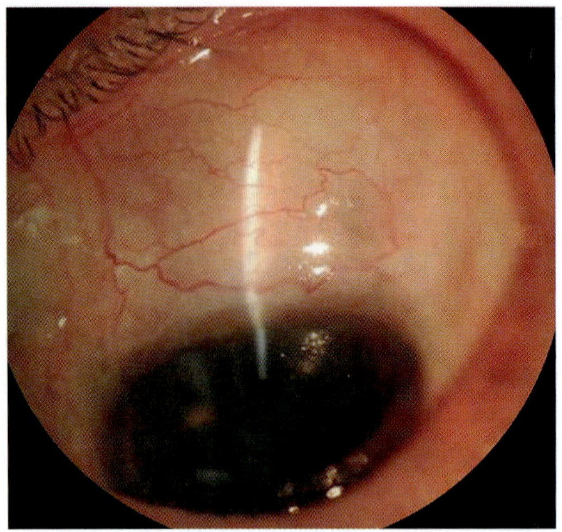

Fig. 20: Good trabeculectomy bleb.

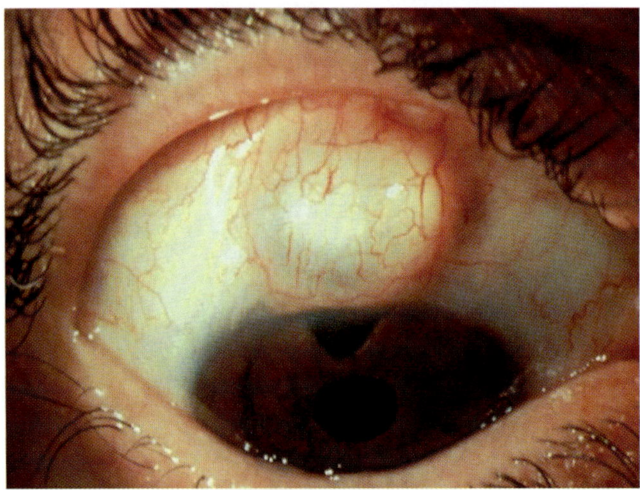

Fig. 21: Tenon's cyst.

The commonly used antifibrotic drugs are injection mitomycin C (MMC) and 5-fluorouracil (5FU). Survival of blebs has now been more predictable, and the earlier complications of avascular blebs and hypotony have now been handled by titrating the doses and the time of exposure.

Aqueous Shunts

All aqueous shunts consist of a tube that diverts aqueous humor to an endplate located under the conjunctiva and Tenon capsule in the equatorial region of the eye. The primary resistance to flow is through these devices, which occur across the fibrous capsule that develops around the endplate.

Aqueous shunts differ in their design with respect to the size, shape, and material composition of the endplate. They may be further subdivided into valved and nonvalved shunts, depending on whether a valve mechanism is present to limit flow through the shunt if the IOP becomes too low. Examples of nonvalved implants are the Baerveldt glaucoma implant, the Aurolab Aqueous Drainage Implant (AADI) implant, the Ahmed ClearPath implant, and the Molteno implant. An example of the valved implants is the Ahmed glaucoma valve **(Figs. 22 and 23)**.

Indications for use of shunts include eyes with neovascular glaucoma, uveitic glaucoma, conjunctival scarring from previous ocular surgery or cicatrizing diseases of the conjunctiva, and congenital glaucoma in which angle surgery has failed. They are used more frequently now and with the

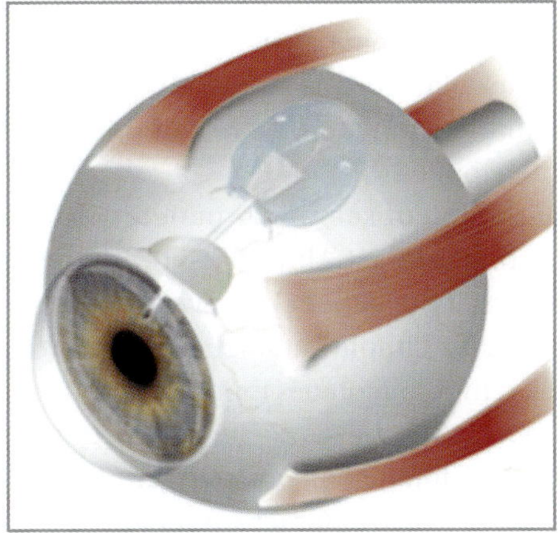

Fig. 22: Ahmed valve.

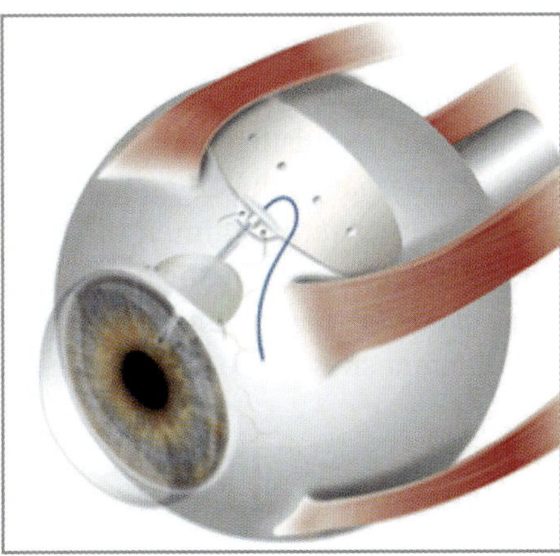

Fig. 23: Baerveldt shunt.

Tube versus Shunt study, where the nonvalved 350 mm^2 Baerveldt was used versus a trabeculectomy as first choice surgery, very promising results have been seen. Tube shunt surgery had a higher success rate than trabeculectomy during 5 years of follow-up, but both surgical procedures were associated with similar IOP reduction, use of supplemental medical therapy, serious complications, and vision loss at 5 years. Shunts with larger surface area endplates have been associated with lower levels of IOP and use of fewer topical ocular hypotensive agents.

Complications of shunts have some things in common with trabeculectomy, but many related specifically to shunts themselves. Tube erosions/endothelial cell loss due to anterior placement of the tube, which can lead to corneal edema and corneal decompensation is mainly due to tube endothelium touch, foreign body reaction, and break down in the blood aqueous barrier resulting in inflammatory mediators. Tube can be blocked by iris, blood, fibrin, and result in rise in IOP. Motility disorders and diplopia can result due to muscular fibrosis or merely from the mass effect of the overhanging bleb on the endplate. The risk of infection is lesser than that seen due to trabeculectomies.

Another unique problem seen with patients having glaucoma is the presence of a coexisting cataract. How to deal with this, is there something that has many answers. If the patient has a well-controlled glaucoma and a significant cataract, just a simple cataract surgery through a clear corneal incision works well. If the glaucoma is mild to moderate and the patient has a significant cataract, again the same surgery works well. However, with the advent of microincisional glaucoma surgery (MIGS), there are plenty of advocates for a MIGS with a cataract surgery in this group. If the patient has an advanced glaucoma and a visually insignificant cataract, it would be worthwhile doing a combined surgery, as doing the cataract surgery later could well land up with a failing bleb. When the cataract is visually significant and the patient has a poorly controlled glaucoma, again the case for a combined cataract surgery with a trabeculectomy is called for. Two-site versus one-site phacoemulsification with trabeculectomy has not shown any advantage of one against the other. But post a trabeculectomy, it is always good to use a long-term regimen of steroids to combat the inflammation and hence help to preserve the functional blebs.

Minimally invasive glaucoma have come to stay and there are multiple procedures targeting different sites in the outflow pathway as described in **Figure 24**.

- *Schlemm's canal:*
    - *Trabecular bypass:* I-stent and high-frequency deep sclerotomy (HFDS)
    - *Schlemm's dilatation:* Hydrus and ab interno canaloplasty

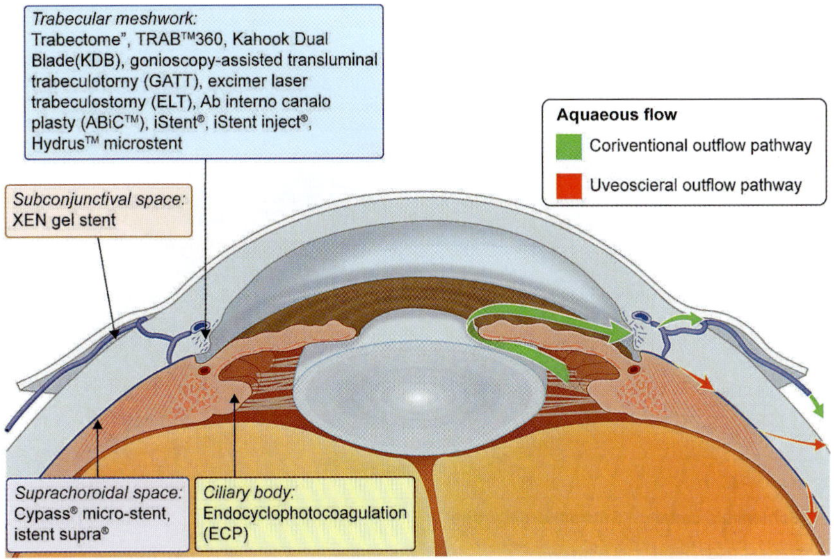

Fig. 24: Schematic of MIGS grouped by mechanism of action.

  - *Trabeculotomy*: Gonioscopy-assisted transluminal trabeculotomy (GATT), bent ab interno needle goniectomy (BANG), Trabectome, Kahook Dual Blade (KDB), and excimer laser trabeculotomy
- *Suprachoroidal space:* CyPass which has been withdrawn.
- *Subconjunctival space:*
  - Ab interno XEN implant
  - Ab externo: PreserFlo
- *Ciliary body:*
  - Ab interno endocyclophotocoagulation
  - Ab externo: Transscleral photocoagulation

What is special about these surgeries that are minimally invasive, most are ab interno procedures, leaving the conjunctiva naïve, cause minimal trauma, are quite effective and have minimal complications. They are only useful in POAG, as you have to have an access to the TM. They are useful in mild to moderate glaucomas and preserve the conjunctiva from the onslaught of preservatives from medications and the fibrosis from surgery **(Fig. 25)**.

To summarize, catching the POAG early is mandatory by doing a comprehensive eye examination at every consultation. Especially so for patients at risk. Each patient needs a tailor-made treatment be it laser, medications, or surgery. The important thing about all glaucomas is to impress the need for a regular follow-up as and when required, as it is a progressive disease and what seems in control at one point of time may progress due to other aggravating factors, like a new comorbidity setting in, or

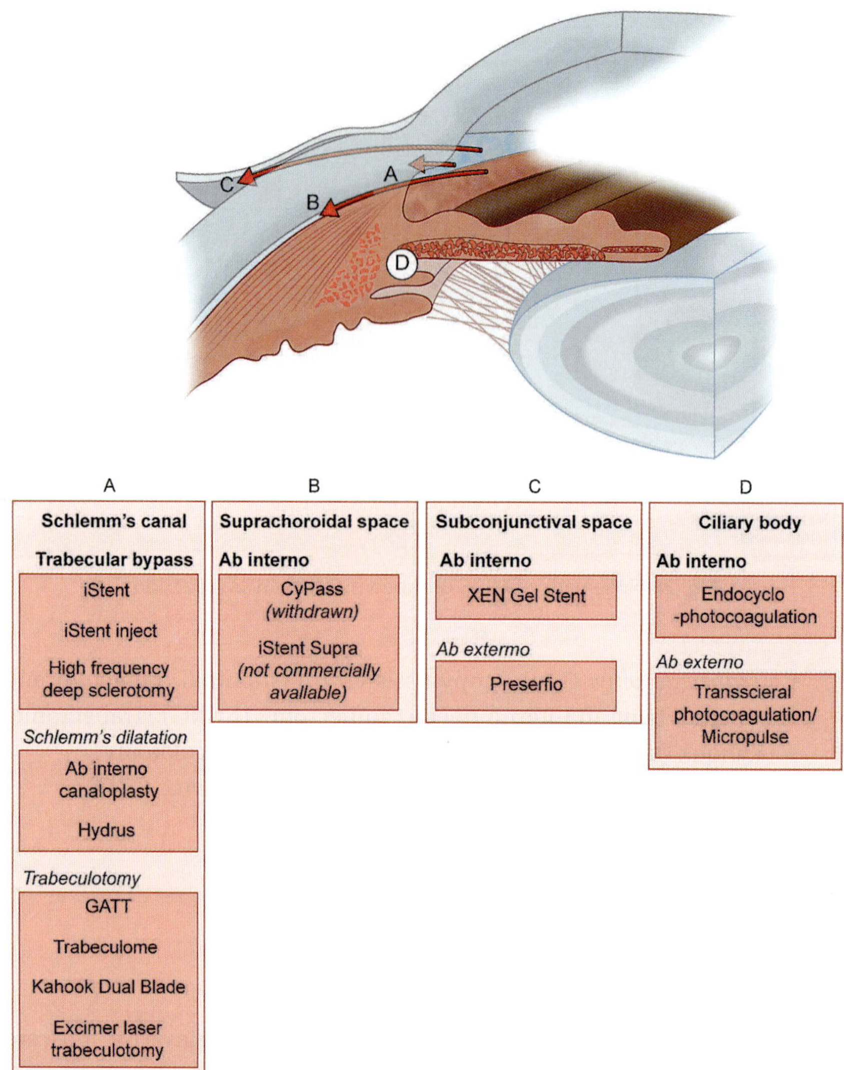

Fig. 25: Subconjunctival space aces where microincisional glaucoma surgery (MIGS) can act (A) Schlemm's canal (B) Suprachoroidal space, (C) Subconjunctival space; (D) The ciliary body.

increasing age and noncompliance. To prevent the patient from going blind, regular monitoring is a very important point to remember.

SUGGESTED READING

1. Allingham RR, Damji KF, Freedman S, Moroi SE, Rhee DJ, Shields MB. Shields' Textbook of Glaucoma. Philadelphia: Wolters Kluwer Health: Lippincott Williams and Wilkins; 2011.

2. Biggerstaff KS. (2024). Primary Open-Angle Glaucoma (POAG). [online] Available from https://emedicine.medscape.com/article/1206147-overview?form=fpf [Last accessed April, 2025].
3. Brandt JD, Beiser JA, Gordon MO, Kass MA; Ocular Hypertension Treatment Study (OHTS) Group. Central corneal thickness and measured IOP response to topical ocular hypotensive medication in the Ocular Hypertension Treatment Study. Am J Ophthalmol. 2004;138(5):717-22.
4. Gedde SJ, Feuer WJ, Lim KS, Barton K, Goyal S, Ahmed II, et al. Treatment Outcomes in the Primary Tube Versus Trabeculectomy Study after 5 Years of Follow-up. Ophthalmology. 2022;129 (12):1344-56.
5. Gedde SJ, Vinod K, Wright MM, Muir KW, Lind JT, Chen PP, et al. Primary Open-Angle Glaucoma Preferred Practice Pattern®. Ophthalmology. 2021;128 (1):P71-P150.
6. Rao HL, Kumar AU, Babu JG, Senthil S, Garudadri CS. Relationship between Severity of Visual Field Loss at Presentation and Rate of Visual Field Progression in Glaucoma. Ophthalmology. 2011;118(2):249-53.
7. Rhee DJ. Glaucoma. In: Porter RE (Eds). The Merck Manual of Diagnosis and Therapy. Rahway, NJ: Merck & Co Inc; 2023.
8. Rivera JL, Bell NP, Feldman RM. Risk factors for primary open angle glaucoma progression: what we know and what we need to know. Curr Opin Ophthalmol. 2008;19(2):102-6.
9. Stamper RL, Lieberman MF, Drake MV. Becker-Shaffers Diagnosis and Therapy of the Glaucomas, 7th edition. Philadelphia: Mosby, an imprint of Elsevier Inc.; 2009.
10. Van Buskirk EM, Cioffi GA. Glaucomatous optic neuropathy. Am J Ophthalmol. 1992;113(4):447-52.

CHAPTER

Secondary Glaucoma

Medha Prabhudesai

INTRODUCTION

Secondary glaucoma is a self-explanatory condition, where there exists a glaucomatous optic neuropathy with a rise in the intraocular pressure (IOP), due to some other existing medical condition, which could be ocular or systemic that is the cause for the glaucoma. Again, secondary glaucoma like their primary counterparts can be either open angle or closed angles depending on the nature of the angle of the anterior chamber (AC).

What are these conditions that can result in secondary glaucomas?

- *Lens-related secondary glaucoma* which could be phacomorphic and phacolytic, especially seen in hypermature cataracts. There could be subluxated/dislocated lenses, resulting in angle closure, misplaced intraocular lenses (IOLs) causing uveitis resulting in synechia.
- *Neovascular glaucoma (NVG):* Diabetic retinopathy and central retinal vein occlusion account for nearly two-thirds of patients with NVG.
- *Uveitic glaucoma:* In uveitis, cells and proteins in the AC disturb the normal outflow of aqueous fluid through the trabecular meshwork (TM), causing raised IOP.
- *Traumatic glaucoma* can happen in all stages of ocular trauma right from the time of the injury to years after the trauma if there is an angle recession following the surgery. Mainly, it happens due to the inflammation post-trauma or due to the hyphema post-trauma to chronic inflammation/uveitis, resulting in peripheral anterior synechiae (PAS) and angle closure or posterior synechiae leading to a pupillary block with an iris bombe formation. There can be a 90-day glaucoma due to clogging of the aqueous drainage by the ghost cells after a hyphema and angle recession leading to glaucoma later in life.
- *Pseudoexfoliative glaucoma:* Abnormal accumulation of particles dandruff like in appearance may accumulate in the angle and cause blockage of the drainage angle.
- *Pigmentary glaucoma:* Pigment particles may circulate abnormally in the aqueous fluid, and these in turn may cause blockage at the drainage angle.
- *Drug-induced glaucoma:* There are many drugs known to give rise to IOP. *Steroids* used either topically or systemically over a period of time

are known to give rise to an increase in IOP in some patients who are labeled as steroid responders. These can be given in any form, may be topically as in allergic conjunctivitis, systemically in systemic diseases like autoimmune disorders, as inhalation therapy in chronic obstructive pulmonary disease (COPD), and as skin ointments for dermatology problems. All can give rise to a steroid response and result in a high IOP. Some steroids are more potent than others and are higher steroid responders as compared to the less potent ones. History of steroid use is a *must* in every patient who presents as a primary glaucoma, as stopping the steroid *is the treatment*, in addition to antiglaucoma medications. Drugs like *topiramate* give rise to a ciliochoroidal effusion and anterior displacement of the lens iris diaphragm giving rise to an acute-angle closure. *Antidepressants* such as selective serotonin reuptake inhibitors (SSRIs) and serotonin-norepinephrine reuptake inhibitors (SNRIs) can cause acute angle-closure glaucoma (AACG). *Antihistamines* such as diphenhydramine (Benadryl), loratadine (Claritin), fexofenadine (Allegra), and cetirizine (Zyrtec) can worsen glaucoma. Cold and flu remedies containing antihistamines or decongestants can worsen glaucoma. Other drugs like *ephedrine* can cause acute angle-closure glaucoma attacks. *Sulfa-based* drugs such as acetazolamide (Diamox) and trimethoprim-sulfamethoxazole (Bactrim) can cause glaucoma. *Anticancer medications* such as docetaxel and paclitaxel can cause glaucoma.

- *Uveitis-glaucoma-hyphema (UGH) syndrome* is a relatively rare clinical condition characterized by chronic postoperative inflammation, high IOP, and hyphema in the AC of an eye post-cataract surgery with IOL implantation.

NEOVASCULAR GLAUCOMA

Neovascular glaucoma is a secondary glaucoma due to neovascularization of the iris and/or AC angle with increased intraocular (IO). There is proliferation of fibrovascular tissue in angle with progressive closure of the angle.

Most common is severe profound retinal ischemia. The incidence is more in patients of central retinal vein occlusion (CRVO) followed by proliferative diabetic retinopathy (PDR) and in ocular ischemic syndrome.

Retinal hypoxia-ischemia increases the production of multiple factors: Vascular endothelial growth factor, nitric oxide, inflammatory cytokines, free radicals, and accumulation of intracellular glutamate.

Pathophysiology

Tiny red nubbins or nonradial, irregular surface capillaries develop adjacent to pupil or iris defects. New vessels have increased permeability. Fibrovascular membrane erupts from peripapillary capillaries and covers the iris surface.

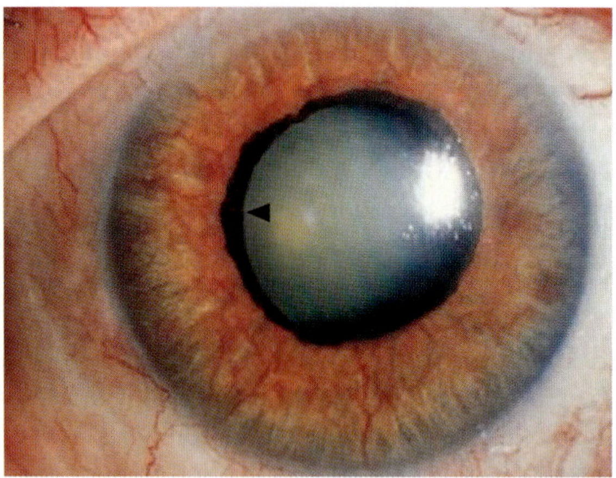

Fig. 1: Ectropion uvea.

It grows toward angle and obstructs the TM causing PAS formation and progressive angle closure. Contraction of the membrane occurs results in ectropion uveae **(Fig. 1)**.

Various stages of NVG can be seen clinically:

- *Early stage of secondary open-angle glaucoma:*
    - Raised IOP
    - Neovascularization of the angle (NVA)
    - Fibrovascular membrane blocks the angle but invisible on gonioscopy
- *Late stage of synechial angle-closure glaucoma:*
    - Fibrovascular membrane contracts forming PAS
    - PAS coalesce to form synechial angle closure
- *Advanced stage:*
    - Fibrovascular resurfacing of cornea
    - Vascularization along lens capsule
    - Formation of cyclitic membrane

Management

Most cases are refractory to medical treatment. For moderate rise in IOP, aqueous suppressants are useful as the angle is closed. Anticholinergics are avoided as they increase inflammation and worsen synechial closure. Prostaglandins are not effective as presence of synechiae and limit the flow of aqueous via the uveoscleral pathway. Cycloplegics and topical steroids are useful to control the inflammation, especially in advanced stage of NVG.

Patient may report with very high IOP. This acute crisis needs to be managed by oral acetazolamide and IV mannitol. Sometimes even paracentesis is needed to control the pain and to reduce the IOP.

There is need to identify retinal pathology leading to ischemia. Early recognition of those at risk helps in salvaging the eye. Anti-vascular endothelial growth factors (anti-VEGFs) can be given to control the neovascularization. In patients with retinal ischemia, panretinal photocoagulation is effective in inhibiting and even reversing neovascularization (NV) proliferation in the anterior segment.

There is no general consensus regarding the best surgical approach for NVG, but the most common surgical approaches are trabeculectomy with antimetabolites or valve implantation preceded by anti-VEGF injections at least a couple of days before the procedure.

Other treatment modalities in the form of endoscopic cyclophotocoagulation, or transscleral diode laser may be needed depending upon stage of the disease and visual potential of the eye.

ANGLE RECESSION GLAUCOMA

Angle recession glaucoma (ARG) is a secondary open-angle glaucoma that is associated with ocular blunt trauma. It is a most common cause of unilateral glaucoma. Many times, the trauma can be unnoticed. It can develop as late as 50 years after blunt trauma.

Incidence of angle recession is 20–90% of eyes after blunt trauma. Development of glaucoma in presence of angle recession is seen in 1–20% of eyes. This depends on extent of angle recession.

If the angle recession is >180°, glaucoma develops in 4–9% whereas if the recession is >240°, incidence is higher.

Angle recession is defined as a tear between the longitudinal and circular layers of the ciliary muscles. Blunt trauma forces aqueous humor laterally and posteriorly against the iris and angle. This exerts traction on the iris root leading to a tear between the longitudinal and circular muscles of the ciliary body. The trabecular dysfunction due to damage to TM due to scarring decreases the outflow of aqueous, leading to increase IOP over time. The other mechanism is damage to the ciliary muscle. This leads to loss of tension on ciliary muscles resulting in narrowing of Schlemm's canal with decreased outflow.

Gonioscopy is the most important clinical examination to diagnose angle recession.

Commonly recessed angle is seen in as a widened ciliary body band. There is asymmetry in gonioscopy findings between quadrants and between two eyes. There can be excessive pigmentation.

Other findings include deepened AC in the same quadrant with sphincter tears.

Anterior segment optical coherence tomography (AS-OCT) and ultrasound biomicroscopy (UBM) can aid in the diagnosis of angle recession.

Management

Medical management is indicated to control IOP.

Topical aqueous suppressants are effective to control IOP β-blockers, carbonic anhydrase inhibitors, and α-agonists. Pilocarpine should be avoided as it may cause paradoxical elevation of IOP.

Laser trabeculoplasty: Selective laser trabeculoplasty (SLT) is relatively contraindicated as it can cause further scarring of the angle structures. SLT is associated with risk of IOP spikes.

Surgical management in the form of trabeculectomy with mitomycin C (MMC) or tube implants are indicated if the IOP is not controlled medically.

PSEUDOEXFOLIATION GLAUCOMA

Pseudoexfoliation syndrome (PXFS) is a systemic condition characterized by the deposition of a protein-like material within the anterior segment of the eye most notably on the anterior lens capsule.

It is also termed as "glaucoma capsulare". Initially, it was thought to originate from the lens capsule.

It is distinct from true exfoliation syndrome which is seen in glass blowers where there is schisis of the anterior lens capsule. Immunohistologic and electron microscopic studies show that the pseudoexfoliation (PXF) material is deposited on the lens capsule, angle, and corneal endothelium and it is a product of abnormal extracellular matrix material metabolism.

All patients of PXFS do not develop glaucoma. Incidence of PXFS is 0.2–27% and for PXF glaucoma, it is 0.07–14.2%. Incidence increases with age. In patients between 60 and 69 years, it is 10%, whereas in patients between 80 to 89 years, it is 33%.

Genetic study shows dysfunction of *LOXL1* (lysyl oxidase-like protein 1) gene, which is important for elastin metabolism. Specific mutations of the *LOXL1* gene are strongly associated with the development of PXF and secondary glaucoma. The defect in elastin metabolism results in synthesis of pseudoexfoliative material.

There can be systemic involvement in the form of impaired regulation of cardiac function. Also, there can be association of vascular diseases and raised homocysteine levels are found in these patients.

Glaucoma due to PXF is secondary open-angle glaucoma due to obstruction of the TM by PXF. Secondary angle-closure glaucoma can be seen in some patients as a consequence of angle closure associated with zonular laxity along with phacodonesis and iridodonesis. This results in forward shifting of iris and lens. Also, there can be iridolenticular adhesions secondary to presence of PXF material.

Clinical Findings

Cornea

There is a decrease in endothelial cell density. Sometimes, corneal guttata is seen which can be secondary to intermittent periods of elevated IOP resulting in cumulative damage to the endothelium. There is deposition of PXF material on endothelium. Pigment dispersion on the endothelium is observed due to disruption of iris pigment epithelium (IPE) due to friction between iris and PXF on the lens capsule.

Anterior Chamber and Iris

Pseudoexfoliation material is seen in AC and on anterior and posterior surface of iris, and on pupillary margin. Transillumination defects can be seen due to atrophic and or fibrotic changes in the iris sphincter muscle. There is loss of the pupillary ruff with appearance of moth-eaten pupil margin.

On gonioscopy, flakes of PXF in the angle are visible inferiorly. Increased but irregular pigmentation in the form of Sampaolesi's line is seen similar to pigment dispersion syndrome (PDS).

Lens

Deposition of flakes of PXF material on the anterior lens capsule is seen as three distinct zones. Central zone of material deposition, clear intermediate zone, which is secondary to iris excursion rubbing the PXF material off of the lens capsule, and third peripheral zone, outside intermediate zone, which can be observed only with dilation.

Zonules laxity results in phacodonesis and forward shifting of lens. PXF zonulopathy is due to the PXF material which indirectly or directly leads to zonular fragility.

Optic Nerve

There is underlying intrinsic increased susceptibility of the optic nerve possibly due to altered extracellular matrix in the nerve head which is associated with decreased structural integrity. There is glaucomatous damage to the optic nerve depending on duration and severity of raised IOP.

Management

Pseudoexfoliation glaucoma is more difficult glaucoma to treat than primary open-angle glaucoma (POAG). There is higher incidence of progression and more likely to be recalcitrant to medical management. Initial medical management effective with most of the antiglaucoma molecules. Prostaglandins are effective in reducing IOP and also in reduction in IOP spikes/diurnal variation. Pilocarpine is not recommended as it may cause development of posterior synechiae and anterior rotation of lens.

Selective laser trabeculoplasty has short-term effect. Post-laser, there can be IOP spikes and increase in inflammation.

Proportion of PXF glaucoma patients undergoing surgical treatment is as high as 87.8%.

Trabeculectomy with or without MMC and valve implants have similar IOP reduction. There can be inflammatory response post-surgery with high risk of bleb failure. More aggressive treatment with steroids is needed for longer period of time and close monitoring is necessary.

PIGMENT DISPERSION SYNDROME AND GLAUCOMA

Pigment dispersion syndrome and glaucoma are characterized by disruption of IPE with deposition of pigment granules on the structures of the anterior segment. There is pigment accumulation in the TM which leads to progressive TM dysfunction resulting in raised IOP with or without glaucomatous optic neuropathy (GON).

It is an autosomal dominant disorder with incomplete penetration. One genetic locus on chromosome band 7q35 has been identified. Risk factors for phenotype expression are myopia and male gender.

Pigment dispersion syndrome is bilateral, seen in younger individuals usually in the third or fourth decade. It typically affects myopes. PDS has 25–50% risk of developing glaucoma. It is more common in men than women (3:1).

Etiology is unknown. There is postulation of abiotrophy, defects of the IPE contribute to their rupture. Histopathological and electron microscope studies have shown that the location of the iris defects closely corresponds to the position of the zonular insertion on anterior lens surface. Also, these patients have posterior iris insertion into the ciliary body (CB), they have concave iris and the IPE is in closer proximity to the zonules. This iridozonular contact leads to increase in iridozonular contact and pigment dispersion. More pigment liberation is seen in eyes with more pronounced iris concavity.

Possible mechanisms responsible for the release of pigment from IPE are friction between iris and anterior lens surface and reverse pupillary block. Pupillary movements cause mechanical rubbing of IPE. Strenuous exercise involving jarring movements, such as jogging or basketball can cause more friction resulting in pigment release. Pharmacologic pupillary dilation results in marked pigment liberation and is accompanied by rise in IOP.

Clinical Findings

The diagnostic triad for PDS is Krukenberg spindle, iris transillumination defects, and dense trabecular pigmentation.

Krukenberg spindle is a vertical accumulation of pigment granules along the corneal endothelium forming a central, vertical, and brown band which is approximately 6 mm long and 3 mm wide. It is slightly decentered inferiorly, wider at its base than its apex. As the age advances, it becomes smaller and lighter and often requires careful examination.

Iris transillumination defects is a classic finding of PDS. The defects are slit-like, radial, and midperipheral. They are best visualized prior to pupillary dilation using a small slit beam in a darkened room.

Pigmentation on TM is called "mascara line". This is seen as a homogeneous, densely pigmented band. *Zentmayer* ring or *Scheie stripe* is pigment accumulation at the zonular attachments to the lens, where it may form a ring. *Egger's line* is deposition of pigment on the anterior hyaloid capsular ligament.

Ultrasound biomicroscopy and AS-OCT can be done to document posterior iris insertion, iris concavity, iridozonular contact, and iridolenticular contact.

With aging, these signs may become very subtle. There is decrease in iridozonular contact with reduction in active pigment release. TM begins to recover and pigment gradually clears. Continued phagocytosis of existing pigment in the TM leads to resolution of pigment in TM. This leads to better aqueous outflow with improvement in IOP control. The pigment band may become darker superiorly more than inferiorly known as pigment reversal sign. This stage is called "burnt-out pigmentary glaucoma" and may be misdiagnosed to have POAG or normal-tension glaucoma (NTG).

Management

Miotics are ideal as they stretch the iris, decrease posterior bowing of iris, and reduce the amount of contact between the iris and the zonules. Prostaglandins are effective but long-term use may exacerbate condition by increasing iris pigmentation. Aqueous suppressants may reduce the IOP, but they decrease the rate of clearance of pigment from TM.

Selective laser trabeculoplasty may be relatively contraindicated. As the TM is heavily pigmented, there can be significant post-SLT elevations in IOP. Laser peripheral iridotomy (LPI) eliminates reverse pupillary block in early stages but is not useful in later stages with raised IOP and damaged TM.

Surgery in the form of trabeculectomy is indicated in patients with uncontrolled IOP. Postoperative hypotony is more common in these patients due to high myopia. These patients are usually in a younger age group with more intense fibrovascular response.

UVEITIS-GLAUCOMA-HYPHEMA SYNDROME

Uveitis-glaucoma-hyphema (UGH) syndrome is a relatively rare clinical condition, usually seen post-cataract surgery with IOL implantation. The syndrome can develop immediately after surgery or over the years.

There is usually a characteristic triad which consists of presence of uveitis, raised IOP, and recurrent hyphema. It is also known as "Ellingson syndrome". Different variants of incomplete UGH syndrome with same etiology can be seen clinically.

Uveitis-glaucoma-hyphema plus syndrome is seen when there is UGH along with vitreous hemorrhage. This is seen with AC IOLs, iris support IOLs, or sulcus fixated IOLs, as there is communication between the vitreous cavity and the AC.

Incomplete posterior UGH (IPUGH) syndrome is noted when there is hemorrhage between the IOL and the posterior capsule, similar to endocapsular hematoma or "in-the-bag hyphema" without uveitis.

In the past, UGH syndrome was mainly seen with older IOLs due to imperfect manufacturing, imperfectly positioned lenses, or improperly sized lenses. It was commonly seen with flexible closed-loop AC IOLs and iris-supported IOLs with metal loops. This was due to design and manufacturing problems, causing sharp edges, vaulting, excess movements, and irritation of ocular tissue.

Presently though UGH syndrome is rare, it is still seen in patients with unconventional use of IOLs like implantation of single-piece foldable acrylic IOLs in the sulcus, or implantation of a single-piece polymethylmethacrylate (PMMA) lens in the bag. Also, it can be seen in patients with scleral fixated IOLs. Formation of *Soemmering ring* cataract can cause anterior shift of sulcus-fixated IOL, leading to iris-haptic touch.

Other mechanisms include the use of surgical devices which can source of mechanical irritation such as iris implants, capsular tension rings, and glaucoma filtration devices.

Patients with PXFS are at higher risk of development of UGH. Pseudophacodonesis due to zonular laxity in these patients can cause chafing of the posterior iris surface. In patients with plateau iris syndrome, haptic in the sulcus can come in contact with anteriorly rotated ciliary processes giving rise to UGH.

The mechanical irritation of the iris, ciliary body, or iridocorneal angle with IOL or any foreign material results in inflammation of these structures. There can be pigment dispersion, hyphema, and sometimes even vitreous hemorrhage. Occasionally, this can be associated with iris neovascularization and cystoid macular edema.

Increase in IOP is mainly due to inflammation and hyphema leading to features of glaucoma.

The inflammation associated with uveitis may directly affect the drainage pathways. Also, there can be mechanical obstruction due to inflammatory cells, proteins, debris, or inflammatory precipitates on the meshwork.

Hyphema can lead to raised IOP. Blood in the AC may obstruct outflow channels with macrophages containing degraded red blood cells and fibrin material.

Management of UGH includes investigations like UBM to find out the cause and investigations for glaucoma mainly OCT for ONH and perimetry.

Medical management includes medications to control anterior segment inflammation to treat cause of recurrent hemorrhage if possible and to lower IOP.

Neodymium-doped yttrium aluminum garnet (Nd:YAG) laser peripheral iridotomy is indicated for sulcus-placed PC IOLs if there is reverse pupillary block. Laser iridoplasty can be done for glaucoma drainage device (GDD) placed near iris. Rarely, frequency-doubled Nd:YAG laser can be done around iris blood vessel if it is seen as a source of recurrent hemorrhage.

There is no "ideal" surgery for UGH at present. Surgery may be indicated to reposition or fixate unstable IOL and in patients with refractory glaucoma to control the IOP.

CHAPTER 11

Comprehensive Guidelines for Medical Management of Glaucoma

Shefali R Parikh, Rajul S Parikh

INTRODUCTION

With the introduction of newer medications in the armamentarium of glaucoma management and diagnostic tools for early diagnosis of glaucoma, decision making in diagnosis, and treatment of glaucoma has become more complex. In this chapter, we describe evidence-based approach to medical management, which we follow in our day-to-day glaucoma practice.

The philosophy of glaucoma management is to preserve the visual function and quality of life (QOL) of the individual patient. Essentially, (functional) vision should outlast the patient. Our aim is not to treat just the IOP, optic disc, or visual field, but to treat patient as a whole so as to provide maximum benefit with minimal side effects.

PRINCIPLES OF GLAUCOMA MANAGEMENT

The basic principles that we follow in the management of a glaucoma patient are discussed below.

- Establish a diagnosis
- Establish a baseline intraocular pressure (IOP)
- Set a target IOP
- Initiate therapy and lower IOP to target
- Follow-up

Establish a Diagnosis

- Careful initial assessment is mandatory to establish the correct diagnosis and to build report with your patient.
- Initial assessment comprises proper history taking and comprehensive eye examination.

History

It is very important to take detailed medical history. Presence of the following systemic disease can affect the disease management directly or indirectly:

- Cardiovascular disease
- Vasospastic diseases

- Hemodynamic crises
- Endocrine diseases
- Sleep apnea disorder

Few systemic and ocular medications can also affect the IOP. For example, steroid administered in any form can cause an increase in IOP.

Steps of Comprehensive Eye Examination

1. Applanation tonometry
2. Gonioscopy
3. Optic disc and retinal nerve fiber layer (RNFL) examination with stereobiomicroscopy
4. Central corneal thickness (CCT) measurement
5. *Automated perimetry*: White-on-white perimetry (WWP)
6. Optic disc and RNFL imaging techniques (optional)

   Flowchart 1 shows a workup of a suspected glaucoma patient in our clinic.

It is important to remember that temporal progression of findings compared to the baseline values (increase in baseline IOP, disc changes, field and imaging parameters), even if they remain within the normal range, can be suggestive of early disease.

Establish a Good Baseline Intraocular Pressure

- IOP is the only known causal and treatable risk factor in glaucoma patient.
- A one-time IOP recording is likely to be misleading; knowledge of diurnal variation of IOP in an individual provides information about the peak IOP as well as fluctuation. It helps to set the target IOP and decide on the group of drugs to be used to initiate treatment.
- Diurnal IOP fluctuation of 8 mm Hg or more on diurnal fluctuation test (DFT) is an independent risk factor for glaucoma progression.
- We usually obtain 24 hours diurnal variation test (DVT) at least in all suspected normal-tension glaucoma (NTG) patients (CCT corrected) and those who are progressing despite "well-controlled" office hours IOP.

Set a target Intraocular Pressure

- The concept of a target IOP recognizes that IOP reduction is a goal of glaucoma therapy.
- Target IOP is not a fixed or a magical digit, but it is a customized range based on patient's clinical profile and glaucomatologist's experienced guess. It is a range below that chances of patient going blind would be minimized.

Flowchart 1: Workup of glaucoma suspect.

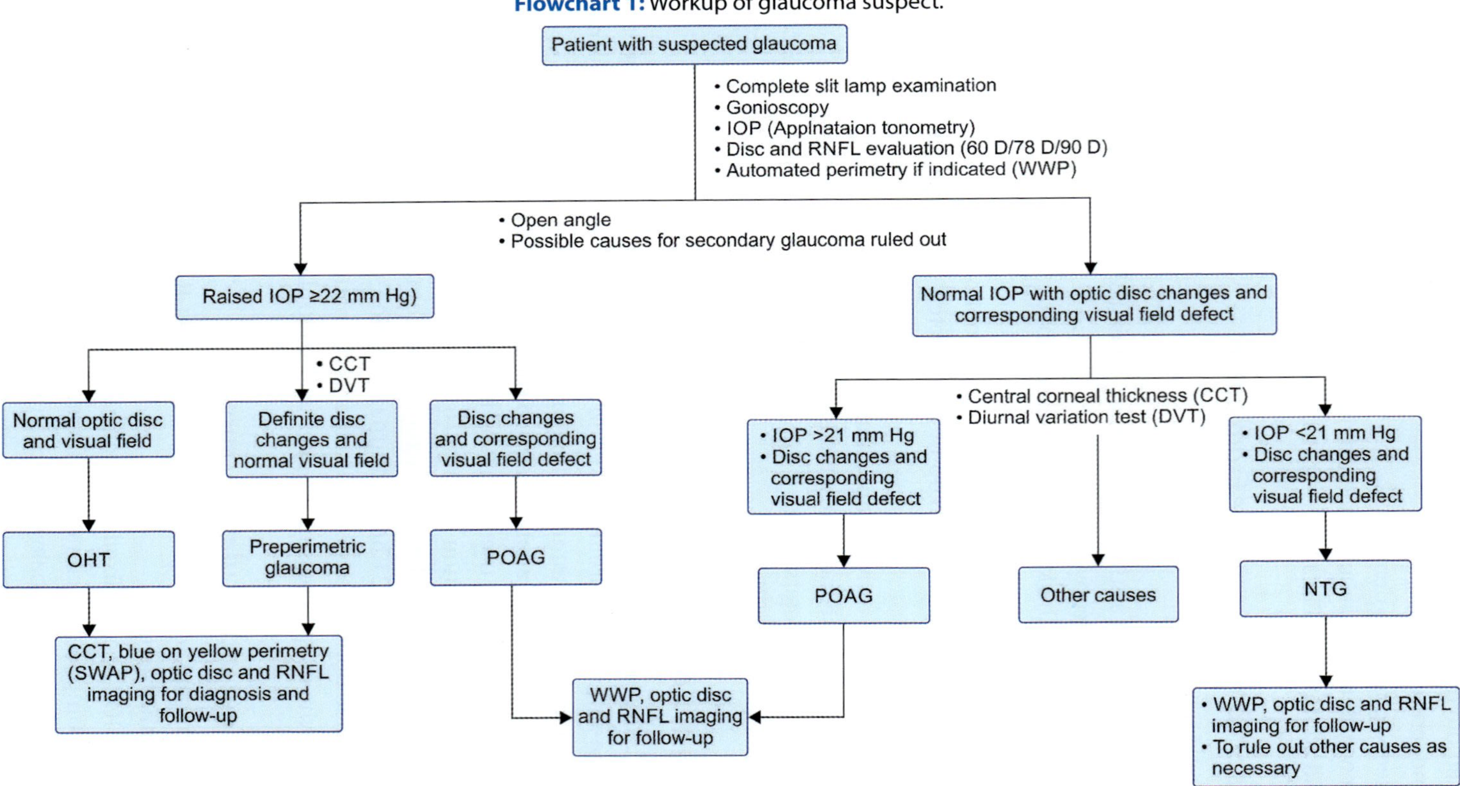

(D: Diopter; IOP: Intraocular pressure; NTG: normal-tension glaucoma; OHT: ocular hypertension; POAG: primary open-angle glaucoma; RNFL: retinal nerve fiber layer; WWP: white-on-white perimetry)

The following factors should be considered to individualize the target IOP:

- The functional and structural damage assessed on WWP and optic disc and RNFL imaging, respectively.
- Baseline IOP at which the damage occurred
- Age of patient: In general, the longer the patient's life expectancy, the lower the target IOP needs to be.
- Presence of additional risk factors like severe damage in the other eye, family history of blindness from glaucoma, etc.

There are various tables and formulas to calculate target IOP. While we can formally calculate this, the rule of thumb is: go on to reduce at least 20% in mild, 30% in moderate glaucoma, and >40% in severe glaucoma [American Academy of Ophthalmology (AAO) guidelines]. The higher the IOP, the more profound percentage reduction will be required. Target IOP is an educated guess. This range of target IOP should be modified, if necessary, rather than adhered to strictly.

Initiate Therapy and Attempt to Lower Intraocular Pressure to Target

- The goal of medical treatment is to obtain "24-hour" IOP control with the minimum concentration and number of medications as well as minimal local and systemic side effects.
- All the antiglaucoma drugs work on two basic principles: (1) reduction of aqueous inflow and (2) increase in aqueous outflow through conventional or unconventional routes. **Table 1** shows the list of available antiglaucoma medications with their mechanism of action and side effects.
- Once initiated, glaucoma therapy is usually lifelong. Accordingly before initiating therapy, we must be sure of the diagnosis, and reasonably sure that the medication works. To establish the efficacy of a drug, we can perform a *unilateral drug trial*. Such a drug trial determines the efficacy of a single or combined therapy in one eye so as to decide if the drug works. The efficacy of the components of a combination must be tested separately.

Flowcharts 2 and 3 show our stepwise treatment ladder what we follow in our practice.

- In an ideal world (not considering cost), we would like to use a prostaglandin (PG) analog in most glaucoma patients as a first line.
- Cost is however a consideration, and if our target IOP is around 20% IOP reduction from the baseline, β-blockers could be the first line of drug. Systemic β-blockers have the ability to achieve 80% of the topical drop's effect on IOP. If the patient is already on systemic β-blockers for hypertension, in such cases, IOP reduction ability of topical β-blockers

TABLE 1: Details of common ocular hypotensive medications.

Drug	*Mechanism of action*	*Duration of action/ daily dosage*	*Systemic side effects, contraindication*	*Local side effects/ contraindication*	*Peak effect and washout period*
• Beta-blockers: Timolol, Levobunolol • Carteolol, Metipranolol • Selective: Betaxolol	Decrease aqueous production	12 hours/twice a day	Bradycardia, hypotension, asthma, bronchospasm, dyspnea, impotence insomnia, hypoglycemia, contraindicated in bronchial asthma, COPD, bradycardia, heart block	Allergic blepharoconjunctivitis, dry eye, corneal anesthesia	4–6 weeks and 4–6 weeks
Miotics *Cholinergics:* • Pilocarpine • Carbachol	Increase trabecular outflow by constricting longitudinal ciliary body muscle and opening trabecular meshwork	6–8 hours four times a day	Increased sweating Salivation, bradycardia	• Miosis, accommodative spasm, iris cysts, anterior subcapsular lens opaciti es, lacrimation • Contraindicated in uveitic, neovascular and lens-induced glaucomas, aqueous misdirection syndrome	Within 3 hours and 1 week
Adrenergics: Adrenaline and dipivefrin	Decrease aqueous production and increase outflow facility	8 hours/three times a day	Headache, nervousness, tachycardia, arrhythmia, hypertension, dry mouth, drowsiness	Mydriasis, lid retraction, adrenochrome deposits, allergic follicular conjunctivitis, CME in aphakia	2 weeks (stabilizes at 6 weeks)

Contd...

Contd...

Drug	***Mechanism of action***	***Duration of action/ daily dosage***	***Systemic side effects, contraindication***	***Local side effects/ contraindication***	***Peak effect and washout period***
• Alpha 2 agonists • Brimonidine • Apraclonidine (not approved for long-term use)	Decrease aqueous production, partially increases uveoscleral outflow	8 hours/three times a day; twice a day if given as combination	Drowsiness, headache, dry mouth, high levels of fatigue, crosses blood–brain barrier, *absolutely contraindicated in patient using MAO inhibitor and <2 years old*	Allergic conjunctivitis	2 weeks (stabilizes at 6 weeks) and 4–6 weeks
Carbonic anhydrase inhibitors (CAIs) *Topical:* • Dorzolamide • Brinzolamide *Systemic*: • Acetazolamide • Methazolamide • Dichlorphenamide	Decrease aqueous production	6–8 hours/three times a day; twice a day if given as combination, systemic CAI 3–4 times a day	Fatigue, malaise, paresthesias of fingers and toes, cramps, diarrhea, nephrolithiasis renal failure, acute leukopenia, agranulocytosis, aplastic anemia, hemolytic anemia, hypokalemia, metabolic acidosis, Stevens–Johnson syndrome	Conjunctival hyperemia, allergic reactions, blepharitis, burning/ stinging sensation, irreversible corneal edema in patients with compromised endothelium (e.g., subclinical Fuchs' dystrophy, post-surgical changes)	72 hours
• Prostaglandin analogs • Latanoprost, travoprost, bimatoprost	Increase uveoscleral outflow	24 hours, once a day	Skin rash, skin pigmentation, iris hyperchromia	Reactivation of herpetic keratitis, cystoid macular edema in pseudophakic and aphakic patients, relatively contraindicated active inflammatory Ocular conditions, CME	2 weeks (stabilizes at 6 weeks) and 6 weeks

Contd...

Contd...

Drug	*Mechanism of action*	*Duration of action/ daily dosage*	*Systemic side effects, contraindication*	*Local side effects/ contraindication*	*Peak effect and washout period*
• Hyperosmotic agents • Mannitol • Oral glycerol	Increase osmolality of blood thus drawing aqueous from vitreous	8 hours	• Caution in patients with cardiac, renal, hepatic disease, nausea and vomiting, circulatory overload—CHF, pulmonary edema, hyponatremia, dehydration, CSF acidosis with poor renal function • Contraindicated in heart failure, pulmonary edema, and renal failure		Mannitol: Peak effect within 1 hour

(CHF: congestive heart failure; CME: cystoid macular edema; COPD: chronic obstructive pulmonary disease; CSF: cerebrospinal fluid; MAO: monoamine oxidase)

Flowchart 2: Stepwise treatment ladder for POAG.

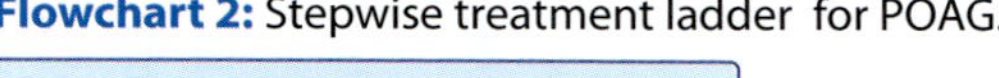

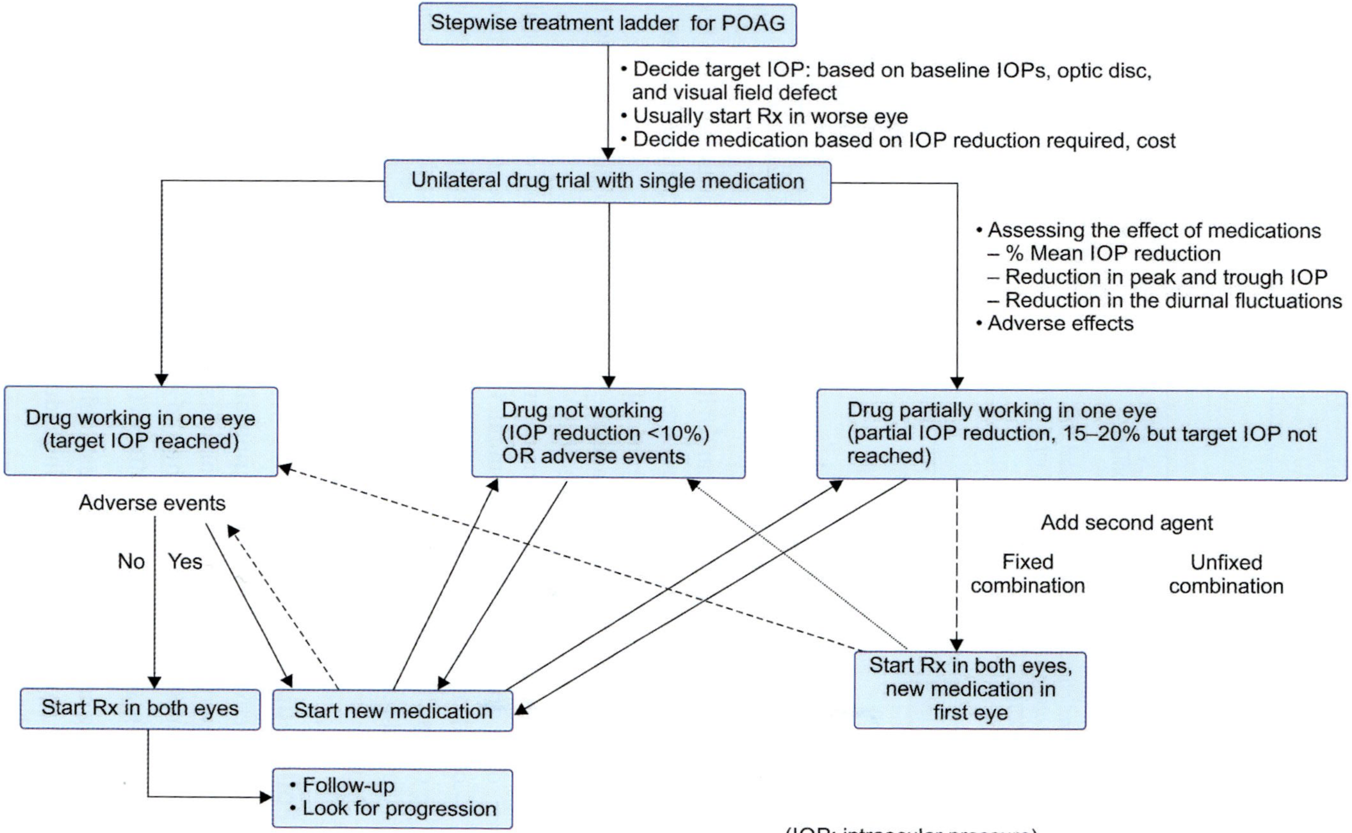

(IOP: intraocular pressure)

Flowchart 3: Topical medical treatment stepladder.

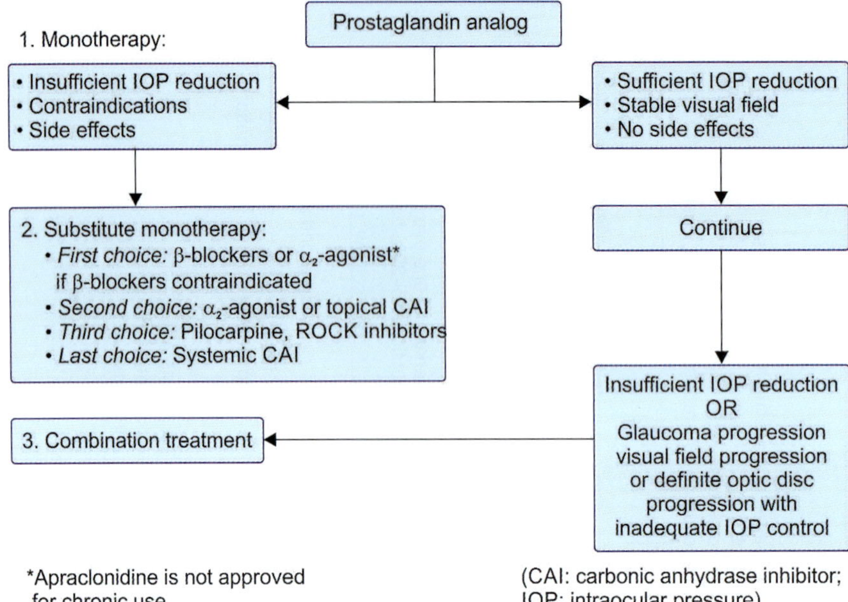

will likely be reduced significantly; it should perhaps be avoided as a first-line drug in this instance. They are, however, worth trying as a second or perhaps third line of management if necessary.

- Combination drugs have made life easier, but each component must be individually shown to be effective.
- While prescribing medications, common side effects and contraindications of the drug should be kept in mind. **Table 1** shows the reported side effects of the common ocular hypotensive medications. Whatever therapy we choose, the concept to be kept in mind is that glaucoma therapy is lifelong and directly related to HRQOL; be its cost, side effects, or regimen of the drug.

Follow-up

The objectives of assessment during follow-up visits are as follows:

- To determine whether glaucoma is stable or progressing.
- If disease is progressing, then to identify underlying mechanism for progression and change treatment (management plan) accordingly.

Following are the factors we must evaluate during follow-up visit. However, we must remember that every individual is unique, and management plan needs to be individualized.

- IOP/target IOP
- Gonioscopy

- Optic disc and RNFL imaging/automated perimetry to judge progression
- Assessing QOL
- Adherence

Progression

- Progression in glaucoma is assessed by structure (optic disc and RNFL) and function (visual field testing with WWP) independently or in association.
- A higher IOP is a risk factor for progression. Structure, function, and IOP should be monitored at regular intervals. The follow-up period depends on the stage of the disease and stability.
- Glaucoma (preperimetric or early functional damage) with IOP at target might be reviewed in 6 months. The yearly follow-ups should include the full comprehensive eye examination as well as several IOPs, visual fields, and other imaging tests required. Stable patients with moderate damage would be examined at 3–4 months intervals. For severe glaucoma in the better eye, the interval could be 2–3 months. **Table 2** shows general guidelines about follow-up, interval for automated perimetry and optic disc examination depending upon initial damage, achievement of target IOP, and progression.

  Some clinical situations' merit has been mentioned below.
- *Normal-tension glaucoma:*
  - Essentially, the approach and treatment are the same as POAG. We only use the term here because it is in common use.
  - Perform a "careful" gonioscopy to rule out primary angle closure (PAC). Do not forget CCT.
  - 24-hour diurnal variation prior to any expensive or invasive investigations. IOP fluctuation of >6–8 is suggestive of IOP-related risk.
  - **Flowchart 4** shows the use for evaluation and follow-up of NTG patient.
  - We may need to look for IOP independent factors such as systemic, nocturnal, orthostatic hypotension, supine IOP rise, sleep apnea syndrome, defective autoregulation, vasospasm/migraine/Raynaud's phenomena, cerebral microvascular disease, and atrial fibrillation
  - Treatment is usually initiated with a PG analog.
  - Certain NTG cases, those with unilateral disease, pallor of the disc, atypical defect, and color defects require appropriate cardiovascular or neurological investigation.
- *Primary angle-closure glaucoma:* The first line of management for chronic primary angle-closure glaucoma (PACG) is laser iridotomy. The details of other laser and surgical options for PACG are out of the scope of this manuscript but a few important points are highlighted:

TABLE 2: General guidelines about glaucoma follow-up depending upon initial damage, achievement of target IOP, and progression.

Target	*Progression*	*Disease status*	*Duration (months)*	*Follow-up (months)*	*Optic nerve Xn*	*Visual field*
Yes	No	Early/moderate	<6	Within 6	6–12 months	5–6 fields in first 2 years and subsequently once a year if disease stable
Yes	No	Advanced	<6	Within 3	6–12 months	5–6 fields in first 2 years and subsequently once a year if disease stable
Yes	No	Early/moderate	>12	Within 6	6–12 months	Once a year if disease stable
Yes	No	Advanced	>12	3 months	6–12 months	6–12 months if disease stable
Yes	Yes	Early/moderate	N/A	2–3 months	3–6 months	At least 6 months
Yes	Yes	Advanced	N/A	Within 2 months	3–6 months	At least 6 months
No	Yes/No	Early/moderate	N/A	3 months	3–6 months	At least 6 months
No	Yes/No	Advanced	N/A	Within 2	3 –6 months	At least 6 months

Flowchart 4: Evaluation of patients suspected with NTG.

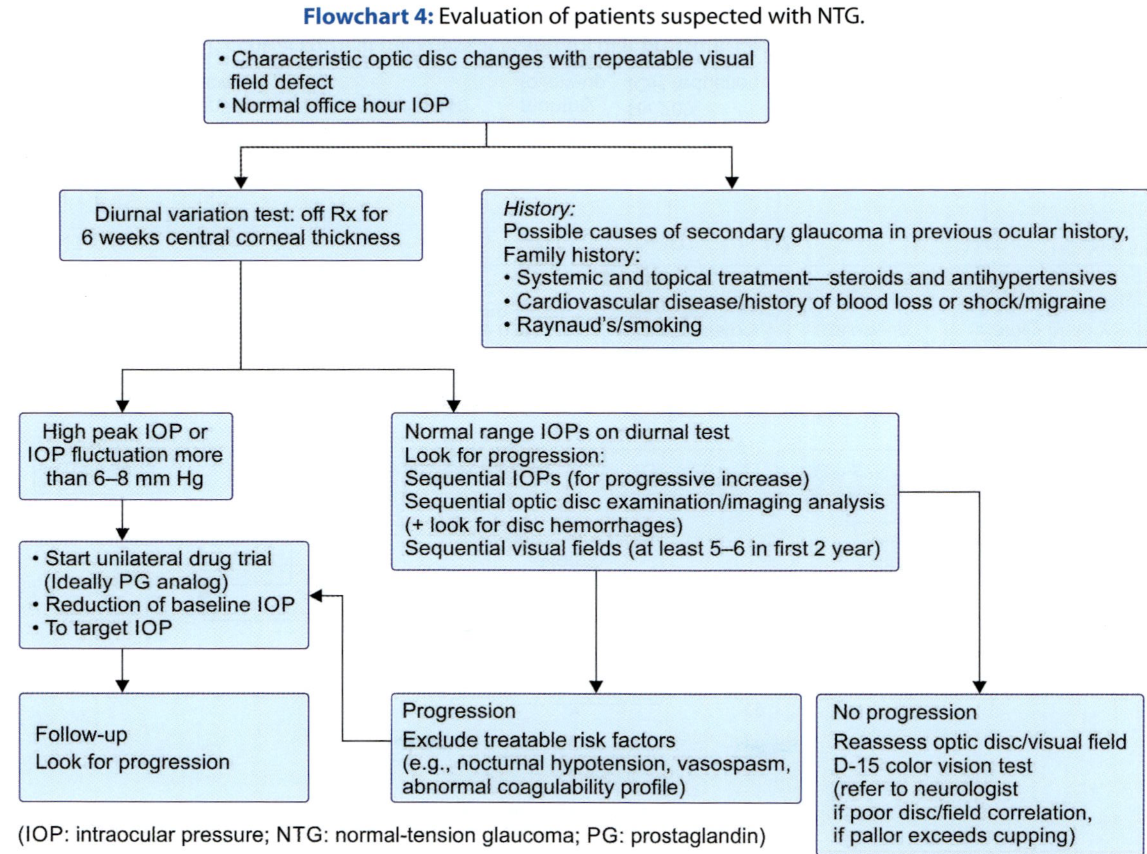

(IOP: intraocular pressure; NTG: normal-tension glaucoma; PG: prostaglandin)

Flowchart 5: Management strategy for OHT.

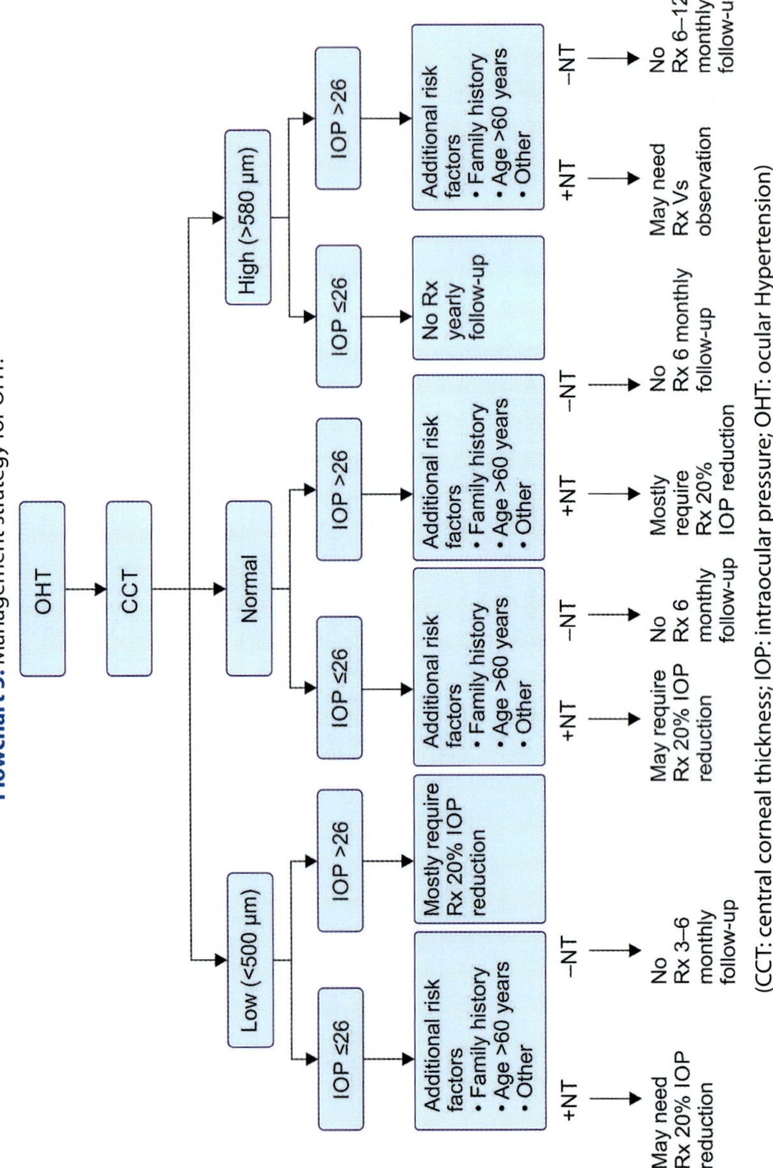

(CCT: central corneal thickness; IOP: intraocular pressure; OHT: ocular Hypertension)

- Laser iridotomy is the first option for chronic PAC or PACG. If fellow eye of PAC or PACG has primary angle-closure suspect (PACS), they should get prophylactic laser peripheral iridotomy.
- Once iridotomy is done and the angle is open in at least 180°, medical management should be same as POAG. If the angle does not open, consider other measures like laser iridoplasty.
- The effect of PG analog is inversely proportional to the degree of closed angle. The effect of PG analog in a totally closed angle is less compared to the effect of PG analog in open-angle glaucoma patients. However, some studies have shown that effect of PG analog in PACG is similar to topical β-blocker and can be tried as a first-line therapy.
- If patient is on pilocarpine for whatever reason, the effect of PG analog on IOP reduction is minimal and other medication (drugs which work on ciliary body) should be used.

- *Ocular hypertension:*
  - Essentially the management is similar to POAG, but the risk of progression is limited. We usually are not as aggressive as POAG patients with functional visual loss.
- Our management philosophy is based on Ocular Hypertension Treatment Study (OHTS) results and other literature like Diagnostic Innovations in Glaucoma Study (DIGS), UCSD, EGPS, and risk calculator based on these studies.
- **Flowchart 5** essentially shows how we manage OHT patients. This flowchart and our management are mainly based on OHTS and other literature.

SUMMARY

Glaucoma is a multifactorial disease and usually is a chronic and slowly progressive disease. At present, all resources are directed toward reduction of IOP, the only known causal and treatable risk factor for glaucoma and medical management are frequently the first choice in most cases. The aim is to prevent any reduction in QOL from visual disability with minimum effects on QOL in terms of cost, side effects, treatment regime, follow-up schedules as well as socioeconomic burden.

SUGGESTED READING

1. Asia-Pacific Glaucoma Society, issuing body. Asia Pacific Glaucoma Guidelines, 3rd edition. Amsterdam, The Netherlands: Kugler Publications, 2016.
2. European Glaucoma Society. Glaucoma guidelines: Terminology and Guidelines for Glaucoma, 3rd edition. Italy: Dogma Publishers; 2009.
3. Parikh RS, Parikh SR, Navin S, Arun E, Thomas R. Practical approach to medical management of glaucoma. Ind J Ophthalmol. 2008;56:223-30.
4. Weinreb RN, Liebmann J, World Glaucoma Association. Consensus series. Medical treatment of glaucoma : the 7th Consensus report of the World Glaucoma Association, 1st edition. Amsterdam: Kugler Publications; 2010.

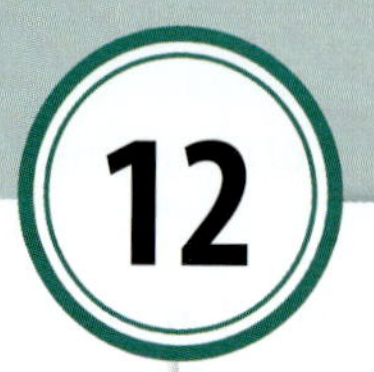

CHAPTER 12

Surgical Management of Glaucoma

Shibal Bhartiya

INTRODUCTION

This chapter delves into the indications, technique, and potential complications associated with trabeculectomy and glaucoma drainage devices (GDDs) providing a comprehensive overview for ophthalmologists, residents, and trainees. It briefly touches upon the common and minimally invasive glaucoma surgeries.

INDICATIONS FOR GLAUCOMA SURGERY

Patients with intraocular pressure (IOP) uncontrolled with maximal tolerated medical therapy (MTMT) and/or lasers; patients who are unsuitable candidates for medical management and/or laser with one or more of the following:

- Progressive optic nerve damage
- Progressive visual field loss
- Expected progression of optic nerve and/or visual field loss due to uncontrolled IOP
- Side effects of glaucoma medication
- Poor compliance with glaucoma medication
- Patients from remote areas with poor access to healthcare, with anticipated loss to follow-up.

CONTRAINDICATIONS FOR GLAUCOMA SURGERY

- Patients with ocular hypertension (OHT) or early glaucoma, with low chances of visual disability
- Short life expectancy
- Systemic conditions precluding safe surgery
- Unwilling patient

TRABECULECTOMY

Trabeculectomy remains one of the cornerstone surgical interventions for managing glaucoma, particularly when medical and laser therapies prove insufficient.

Indications

Patients with glaucoma who have not achieved adequate IOP control with medications or laser treatments.

Technique

The trabeculectomy procedure involves creating a fistula to allow aqueous humor to drain from the anterior chamber to the subconjunctival space, thus lowering IOP. The key steps include:

- *Preoperative preparation:* Ensuring adequate patient consent, administering local anesthesia, and preparing the surgical field.
- *Conjunctival flap creation:* A limbal-based or fornix-based conjunctival flap is fashioned to expose the sclera.
- *Scleral flap creation:* A partial-thickness scleral flap is dissected, typically rectangular or triangular in shape, to facilitate controlled aqueous outflow.
- *Trabecular meshwork excision:* A block of trabecular meshwork and adjacent corneal stroma is excised to create a communication between the anterior chamber and the subconjunctival space.
- *Scleral flap closure:* The scleral flap is sutured loosely to allow for controlled filtration of aqueous humor. Adjustable sutures may be used to fine-tune IOP postoperatively.
- *Conjunctival closure:* The conjunctival flap is meticulously closed to prevent leaks and ensure a well-formed bleb.
- *Postoperative care:* Involves close monitoring, the use of anti-inflammatory and antibiotic eye drops, and managing complications promptly. Mitomycin C (MMC) versus 5-fluorouracil (5FU).

Mitomycin C

- More potent, therefore, lower IOP
- Freshly reconstituted from powder to appropriate concentration by dilution
- Higher incidence of complications
- *Intraoperative use:* 0.2–0.4 mg/mL for 1–3 minutes.

5-fluorouracil

- Inexpensive
- No dilution or dosage calculation
- Stable at room temperature
- Better safety profile
- *Intraoperative use:* 50 mg/mL for 1–5 minutes.

Complications

While trabeculectomy is generally effective, it carries risks of intraoperative and postoperative complications.

Early Complications

- *Hypotony:* Excessively low IOP due to overfiltration, which can lead to choroidal detachment or maculopathy.
- *Shallow or flat anterior chamber:* Requiring urgent intervention to prevent synechiae formation or lens-cornea touch.
- *Bleb leak:* Early or late bleb leaks can lead to hypotony or infection. Managing leaks may involve conservative measures or surgical revision.
- *Infection:* Endophthalmitis and blebitis, although rare, are serious and necessitate prompt antibiotic therapy.

Late Complications

- *Cataract formation:* Trabeculectomy is associated with an increased risk of cataract progression, likely due to surgical trauma and postoperative inflammation.
- *Bleb failure:* Scarring of the bleb can lead to failure, necessitating bleb revision, or alternative glaucoma surgeries.
- *Overhanging bleb:* It may cause discomfort, dellen formation, or dysesthesia. Managing these requires careful surgical revision.
- *Encapsulated bleb:* Excessive scarring around the bleb can limit its function, often requiring needling or antimetabolite injections to restore function.

GLAUCOMA DRAINAGE DEVICES

Glaucoma drainage devices shunt aqueous humor from the anterior chamber to an external reservoir, where a fibrous capsule forms about 4–6 weeks after surgery and regulates aqueous outflow. GDDs are usually used for eyes with previously failed trabeculectomy or eyes with insufficient conjunctiva secondary to scarring from prior surgical procedures. GDDs are available in different sizes, materials, and design with the presence or absence of an IOP regulating valve. The nonvalved options include the Baerveldt glaucoma implant (Advanced Medical Optics, Inc., Santa Ana, CA, USA), Molteno (IOP, Inc., Costa Mesa, CA, USA, and Molteno Ophthalmic Limited, Dunedin, New Zealand), Eagle Vision implants (Eagle Vision, Inc. Memphis, TN, USA), Aurolab aqueous drainage implant (AADI, Aurolab, India), and the recently launched, Paul glaucoma implant (PGI, Advanced Ophthalmic Innovations, Singapore, Republic of Singapore). Most commonly used valved implant is the Ahmed glaucoma valve (AGV) (New World Medical, Rancho Cucamonga, CA, USA).

The decision to choose a particular type of drainage device depends on a patient's underlying characteristics in terms of preoperative IOP and optic nerve status, desired long-term IOP control, and the surgeon's comfort and preference.

Indications

Glaucoma drainage devices are generally used for complicated/refractory as well as secondary glaucomas. They may also be used as primary procedures depending on surgeon preference. The list of indications includes:

- Secondary glaucomas including neovascular, uveitic, traumatic, post-vitreoretinal surgery, post-keratoplasty, and aphakic or pseudophakic
- Refractory congenital or developmental glaucoma
- Anterior chamber dysgenesis including iridocorneal endothelial syndrome
- Severe conjunctival scarring
- Previously failed trabeculectomy.

Valved versus Nonvalved Glaucoma Drainage Devices (Table 1)

Valved GDDs may be preferred in the following cases:

- *Beginner surgeon:* The surgical technique is simpler with localization to one quadrant without manipulation of the adjacent rectus muscles.
- *Early IOP control:* IOP control in the early postoperative period is more predictable because of flow-restricting mechanisms.
- *Patients with poor compliance with postoperative medication use and follow-up visits:* Valved GDDs usually require less postoperative follow-up and care.

Technique

- A fornix-based or limbus-based conjunctival incision is created to allow adequate exposure for insertion of the plate.
- A corneal or scleral suture can be placed to improve exposure in the working quadrant.
- For a nonvalved implant, the implant is anchored between two recti with the anterior edge approximately 8–10 mm posterior to the limbus. Larger implants (Baerveldt) are inserted with the long axis directed toward the apex of the orbit and then rotated horizontally so that the tube points directly toward the anterior chamber and the wings of the implant are under the rectus muscles. Whenever possible, single-plate implants should be placed in the superotemporal quadrant.
- If a two-plate implant is used, one plate is positioned in each of the two quadrants. The tube connecting the two plates may be passed under or over the intervening rectus muscle.
- All valved implants require priming of the tube prior to the plate anchorage. The tube is primed with balanced salt solution with a 30-gauge cannula to open up the valve leaflets. The tube of the nonvalved implant should be irrigated as well to ensure its patency.
- Implant plate is secured to the globe with two nonabsorbable sutures (8-0 or 9-0 nylon sutures on a spatulated needle).

TABLE 1: Commonly used valved and nonvalved glaucoma drainage devices (GDDs).

Valved GDDs			
Type	***Model***	***Size (mm²)***	***Plate material***
Ahmed Glaucoma Valve (AGV)			
Single plate	S2	184	Polypropylene
Pediatric size	S3	96	Polypropylene
Single plate	FP7	184	Silicone
Pediatric size	FP8	96	Silicone
Pars plana	PS2	184	Polypropylene
Pars plana (pediatric)	PS3	96	Polypropylene
Pars plana	PC7	184	Silicone
Pars plana (pediatric)	PC8	96	Silicone
Nonvalved GDDs			
Type	***Model***	***Size***	***Material***
Baerveldt Glaucoma Implant (BGI)			
Single plate	103–250	250	Silicone
Single plate	101–350	350	Silicone
Pars plana	102–350	350	Silicone
Ahmed ClearPath (ACV) Implant			
Single plate	250	250	Silicone
Single plate	350	350	Silicone
Eagle Vision Implant	EG365	365	Silicone
Molteno Implant			
Single plate	S1	137	Polypropylene
Single plate/ridge	D1	137	Polypropylene
Double plate	R2/L2	274	Polypropylene
Double plate/ridge	DR2/DL2	274	Polypropylene
Molteno 3/single plate	GS	175	Polypropylene
Molteno 3/double plate	GL	230	Polypropylene
Aurolab Aqueous Drainage Implant (AADI)			
AADI350/single plate		350	Silicone
AADI250/single plate		350	Silicone
Paul Glaucoma Implant (PGI)			
Single plate	P2015001	342.1	Silicone

- Aqueous drainage through a nonvalved device can be regulated in the early postoperative period by passing a 4-0 Prolene suture through the lumen of the implant. Once the fibrous capsule around the plate has formed, the stent suture is removed at the slit lamp. Alternatively, external occlusion using a suture ligature around the external aspect of the tube can be accomplished using a 7-0 or 8-0 absorbable Vicryl suture.

- After this, the tube is laid over the cornea and cut with sharp scissors to create a bevel up toward the cornea, or with the bevel posteriorly in sulcus positioned tubes. The tube must extend approximately 2.5–3 mm into the anterior chamber.
- A 23-gauge needle is used to create a track through which the tube is inserted into the anterior chamber, anterior and parallel to the iris, or into the sulcus between the iris and lens (in pseudophakes).
- To stabilize the tube, the tube is secured to the sclera a few millimeters anterior to the plate with 7-0 or 8-0 Vicryl suture. This suture should not be too tight.
- Many prefer to cover the tube with a patch graft (sclera or pericardial patch graft), which is secured to the globe with interrupted sutures at the anterior corners using 8-0 nylon sutures. Some surgeons create a partial thickness scleral flap and then create a needle track and insert the tube under this flap. This flap is then sutured with 10-0 nylon sutures.
- The conjunctiva and tenons are pulled over the plate, tube, and patch graft and secured into place with 8-0 Vicryl suture.
- At the end of the procedure, a subconjunctival injection of antibiotic and steroid is given.
- For valved GDDs, preoperative antiglaucoma medications are stopped to prevent hypotony. However for the nonvalved GDDs, the antiglaucoma medications are continued until a fibrous capsule forms around the plate, at that point usually the ligature suture may spontaneously open.

Common Complications

- *IOP related issues:*
  - Hypotony, choroidal effusions or rarely, suprachoroidal hemorrhage, are more commonly observed with the nonvalved GDDs.
  - *Hypertensive phase with IOP:* Ranging from 30 to 50 mm Hg, it may occur anywhere between 1 and 6 weeks postoperatively.
- *Tube-related issues:*
  - Anteriorly placed tube may cause decompensation of the corneal endothelium. On the other hand, if the tube is placed too posteriorly, chronic inflammation may occur due to repeated iris rubbing.
  - If the tube touches the anterior lens capsule, then it may result in cataract formation.
  - Short tubes can retract. Retracted tubes can be lengthened with tube extenders or may be placed in the pars plana.
  - Tube block from blood, vitreous, fibrin, or iris incarceration!
  - Tube erosion may occur.
- *Plate-related issues:*
  - Migration or extrusion of plate may occur.
  - Diplopia or strabismus.

MINIMALLY INVASIVE GLAUCOMA SURGERY

The last decade has witnessed an unprecedented growth in glaucoma treatment options through the introduction of minimally invasive glaucoma surgery (MIGS). The working definition for this rather heterogeneous group of surgeries (as per the American Glaucoma Society) includes surgeries that:

- Lower IOP improving aqueous outflow
- Device or procedure can have either an ab interno or ab externo approach
- Limited surgical manipulation of the sclera and the conjunctiva, and usually not bleb dependent.

Contraindications

The relative contraindication for each specific MIGS is to be evaluated and individualized for each patient. Main contraindications include:

- Angle-closure glaucoma!
- *Secondary glaucoma:* Inflammatory, traumatic, and neovascular
- Advanced glaucoma
- Previous glaucoma surgery
- Very low target IOP
- One-eyed patient

Classification of Minimally Invasive Glaucoma Surgery

The anatomical outflow pathway as well as the surgical approach may be used to classify MIGS.

- *Subconjunctival filtration strategy:*
  - *Ab externo approach*:
    - Carbon dioxide (CO_2) laser-assisted sclerectomy surgery (CLASS)
    - InnFocus MicroShunt
  - *Ab interno approach:* XEN implant
- *Enhanced filtration into synergetic control SC strategy:*
  - *Ab externo approach:*
    - Canaloplasty
    - Stegmann canal expander
  - *Ab interno approach:*
    - iStent
    - High-frequency deep sclerotomy (HFDS)
    - Ab interno trabeculotomy (Trabectome)
    - Hydrus implant
    - Kahook Dual Blade (KDB)
- *Suprachoroidal filtration strategy:*
  - *Ab interno approach:*
    - iStent Supra implant
  - *Ab externo approach:*
    - Starflo implant
    - Gold Solx implant

Focusing on the commonly used MIGS:

- *iStent:* The iStent (Glaukos, Laguna Hills, CA) was approved by the Food and Drug Administration (FDA) in 2012. Currently used models are the iStent infinite® Trabecular Micro-Bypass System Model iS3 and iStent inject® W. The key difference between the iStent infinite® and the iStent inject® W is that the iStent infinite has three preloaded stents within a single injector, while the iStent inject W only has two stents, making the iStent infinite capable of implanting more stents in a single sitting. Stents are inserted along approximately 6 clock hours around Schlemm's canal. It bypasses the trabecular meshwork to create a direct communication between the anterior chamber and Schlemm's canal. It is approved for use at the time of cataract surgery in patients with mild to moderate POAG on 1–3 medications. The iStent G3 Supra is a suprachoroidal stent which is currently being studied for use with concurrent cataract surgery in a multicenter randomized controlled trial.
- *Kahook Dual Blade:* The KDB (New World Medical, Rancho Cucamonga, CA) is a novel ab interno goniotomy device. It allows the surgeon to cleave the trabecular meshwork for approximately 120°. The procedure is akin to the Trabectome procedure, however, it uses a dual-blade scalpel rather than a cautery.
- *Omni:* The OMNI® Surgical System from Sight Sciences, combines a canaloplasty with a trabeculotomy and can be performed with cataract surgery or in pseudophakic patients as an alternative to trabeculectomy. It is the only MIGS device capable of addressing the trabecular meshwork, Schlemm's canal, and the distal collector channels at the same time.
- *Gonio-assisted transluminal trabeculotomy (GATT):* For patients with open-angle glaucoma requiring significant IOP reductions, more robust IOP control can be obtained GATT. It is a form of ab interno trabeculotomy in which an illuminated fiberoptic microcatheter (iScience International, Menlo Park, CA) is advanced circumferentially through Schlemm's canal and then externalized to open the trabecular meshwork for a full 360°. GATT can also be performed after a failed trabeculectomy or GDD. The main adverse event associated with this surgery is postoperative hyphema, which usually resolves on its own.
- *Ab interno canaloplasty:* Ab interno canaloplasty (iTrack, Ellex) involves the viscodilation of Schlemm's canal. This also allows breaking adhesions in the trabecular meshwork and irrigation of the collector channels.
- *Hydrus Microstent:* The Hydrus Microstent (Ivantis Inc, Irvine, CA, USA) is a trabecular bypass stent intended for use at the time of cataract surgery. It is 8 mm in length and has a curved shape to facilitate scaffolding and dilation of Schlemm's canal for 3 clock hours. This is by far the largest-sized MIGS option available. The device covers 90° within the angle.

- *XEN gel stent:* The XEN gel stent (Abbvie) is a collagen implant, 6-mm hydrophilic flexible tube with a 45-μm lumen (XEN45). Stent is implanted with a sterilized, single-hand inserter containing a 27G needle that is preloaded with one gelatin stent. It is inserted ab interno through the scleral spur into the subconjunctival space. The device hydrates within 1–2 minutes of coming in contact with the aqueous humor, conforming to the tissue. The design of the XEN gel stent is based upon the principles of laminar fluid dynamics. The most common complications of this stent include subconjunctival fibrosis requiring bleb needling and transient hypotony.
- *InnFocus Microshunt:* The InnFocus Microshunt is currently under development and not yet FDA approved. It is an aqueous drainage device that is implanted through an ab externo modified filtering procedure. It drains aqueous fluid 3 mm posterior to the limbus to a subconjunctival flap created with adjunctive MMC.

SUGGESTED READING

1. Dhingra D, Bhartiya S. Evaluating glaucoma surgeries in the MIGS context. Rom J Ophthalmol. 2020;64(2):85-95.
2. Khodeiry M, Sayed MS. New glaucoma drainage implants available to glaucoma surgeons. Curr Opin Ophthalmol. 2023;34(2):176-80.
3. Lim R. The surgical management of glaucoma: A review. Clin Exp Ophthalmol. 2022;50(2):213-31.
4. Mathew DJ, Buys YM. Minimally Invasive Glaucoma Surgery: A Critical Appraisal of the Literature. Annu Rev Vis Sci. 2020;6:47-89.
5. Razeghinejad MR, Spaeth GL. A history of the surgical management of glaucoma. Optom Vis Sci. 2011;88(1):E39-47.

CHAPTER 13

Journey of a Glaucoma Patient

Rita Dhamankar

INTRODUCTION

The physician and the patient both have different perspectives of the same disease where glaucoma is concerned. Physicians claim the success of glaucoma management with parameters such as intraocular pressure (IOP), visual fields, and damage progression. However, from the perspective of the patients, other concerns may be far more important. The most frequent problems related to decreased vision were reading, walking on stairs, and recognizing people **(Fig. 1)**.

Glaucoma can be devastating. The most feared impact is sight loss.

There are other wide-ranging systemic, psychological, emotional, and social effects of both the disease and its treatment. Every stage of the disease throws up a new challenge. It is very important to know what the patient feels.

The journey differs from patient to patient, the extent of the disease he has. The journey differs from time to time, and differs from patients with the kind of glaucoma he has. Hence, QOL is so important in the definition of treating glaucoma **(Figs. 2A to C)**.

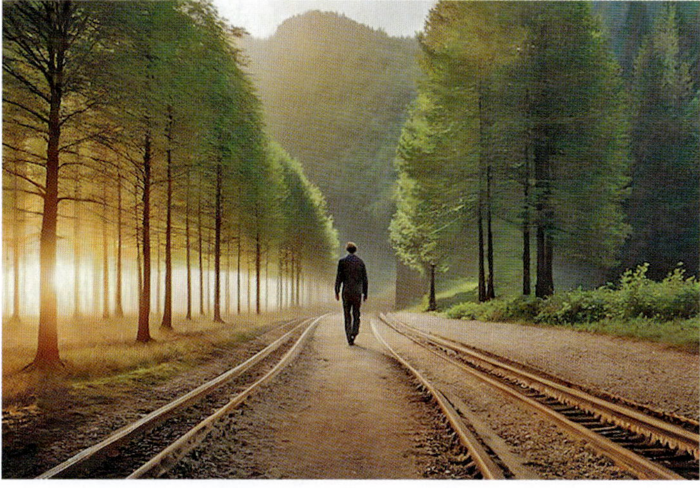

Fig. 1: Depicting a journey.

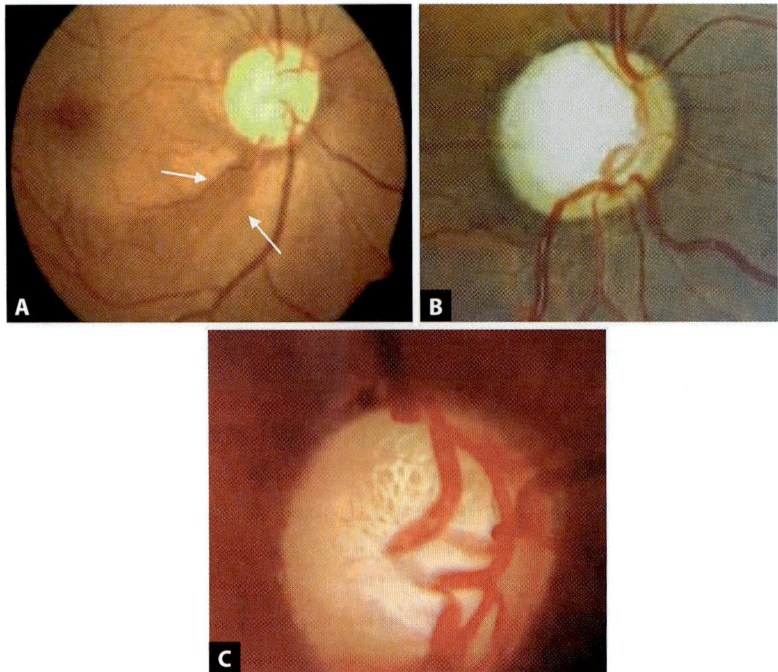

Figs. 2A to C: Early, moderate, and advanced glaucoma.

Each of these patients could be on a different journey depending on their age, their profession, and their personality. So, every patient is to be looked at, as an individual on his own journey **(Fig. 3)**.

Let us look at some real-time situations.

In a patient who comes with an acute angle-closure glaucoma, he comes with acute redness, severe pain, watering, and *loss of vision*. At the onset itself, he is scared, because there is a loss in vision. He is in pain. He wants relief at any cost. He is going to be the most satisfied patient. You can give him a lot of relief. His pain is taken care of. Many times, vision is restored fully. This infuses tremendous confidence in the patient. He is a very satisfied patient. You need to educate him. He needs to remain compliant. As against a patient with an angle-closure disease, who may have headaches specifically in the dark, may have haloes occasionally. He may be completely unaware of the cause. When a diagnosis is shared, he is quite willing for treatment. Counseling for him to be compliant is very important.

Quite to the contrary, a patient with a primary open-angle glaucoma (POAG) is the most difficult patient. He has no symptoms. His diagnosis is de novo. Many times, he has not even heard of the term glaucoma. Sometimes, he has heard that there is no treatment for glaucoma. At first, there is a shock, disbelief, and why me attitude? Early on in the disease, they are reluctant

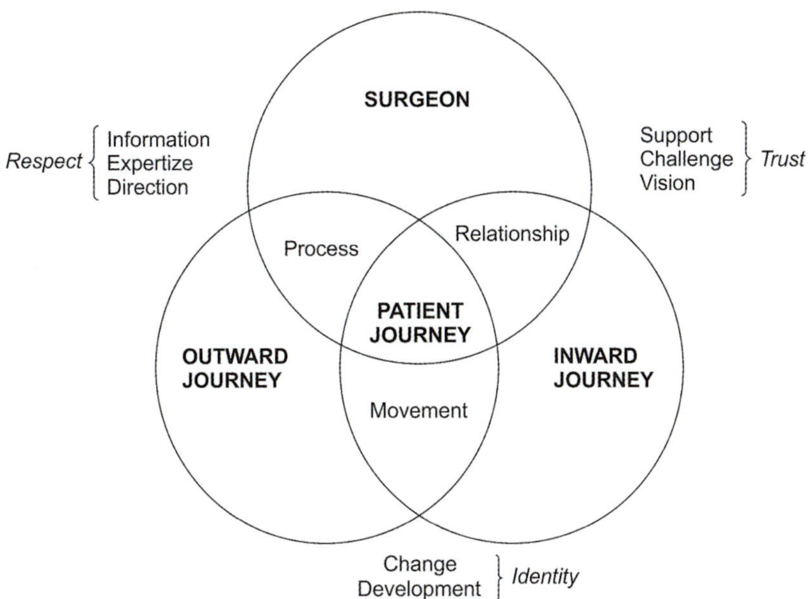

Fig. 3: Depicting what is common between what the surgeon thinks and the patient thinks both externally and inside.

to even get investigations done, they see no need. Later they read, educate themselves, and are now in constant fear of going blind.

"How do you counsel the patient?" is what affects the patient most. Here is a patient with no complaints, and you have added a label. Here, what you do matters most. He is subjected to various repeat tests, which are difficult to do and are expensive too. He cannot make head or tail of that report. He is given medications. The medication costs, hurts, and disturbs his daily schedule. Then, he learns about the progression of the disease. He sees no good from medication. He faces red eyes, itching, burning, and the additional burden of remembering to use the medications timely. As if this was not enough, he has to repeatedly visit his ophthalmologist. There are more tests, more medications, and more counseling sessions.

This can be very demotivating to the patient. This can also be the reason for a poor quality of life, in addition to having poor visual function. Quality of life may be compromised right from the time a diagnosis is made till the time he departs. It is our duty, as treating physicians, to not only ensure that the patient's vision is preserved, but also that he maintains a good quality of life. Always instill hope and no fear in your patients. Be open to discussing what their fears are, what their life demands. Be proactive in offering solutions that you can, to help them overcome fears. It is a very good idea to have a glaucoma club, where you can invite all your patients and give them some important updates in glaucoma that they may be interested in. Let this session be interactive. Get as many people to participate in the interaction as possible. Let the patients interact with one another. Here patients with queries can spend some extra time both with similar patients and you with your counseling team. That gives them a lot of confidence and proves to be very helpful in terms of their compliance as well as follow-ups. Some patients who may have come to you in a very advanced stage, may be absolutely scared of going blind. But meeting other patients who have had advanced disease for long, only makes him happy. Someone who has side effects due to medications, will willingly accept a surgical option/selective laser trabeculoplasty (SLT), once he sees your surgical/SLT results. People will realize how important it is to also involve their caregivers in these meetings, as the caregiver becomes more compassionate and more active in patient care.

Giving them the services of a low vision clinic, certainly helps them maneuver their way through life far more comfortably. They can move about independently, look after their finances by themselves, and engage in activities such as music, reading, listening to good audios, having met people who do this regularly and are not a burden to any of their family members. Pick out all your success stories and get a couple of them to share their stories with the others.

You might also invite some philanthropists to this meeting, as they might be tempted to pay for someone's treatment, if he finds it is worthwhile. Some pharmaceuticals might also like to attend these meetings to talk about the benefits they can give patients regularly ordering medications. They may opt to sponsor some regular investigations.

You could also give them an annual membership, which gives them access to your opinions at a discount and investigations at a discount. Many times, the expense of the treatment is a factor that keeps patients away from treatment as they do not see the benefit of treatment in terms of visual recovery. Every human is lured with freebies, and offering it to a deserving patient goes a long way, in helping them to live a relatively happy life.

They have to be counseled about loss of contrast, and keeping their outside activities limited to the daytime. This will help them go out and socialize, shop, look after their finances, etc. independently. At the same time, never miss an opportunity to tell them how good they are, and how you are happy with their progress, when they are compliant. This response from the treating physician does wonders for the patient's psyche. Never ask a patient directly about how compliant they have been, always ask them how often have they forgotten their medications, so they will always come out with the truth and avoid the white coat syndrome, of using medications, just a couple of days before coming to you.

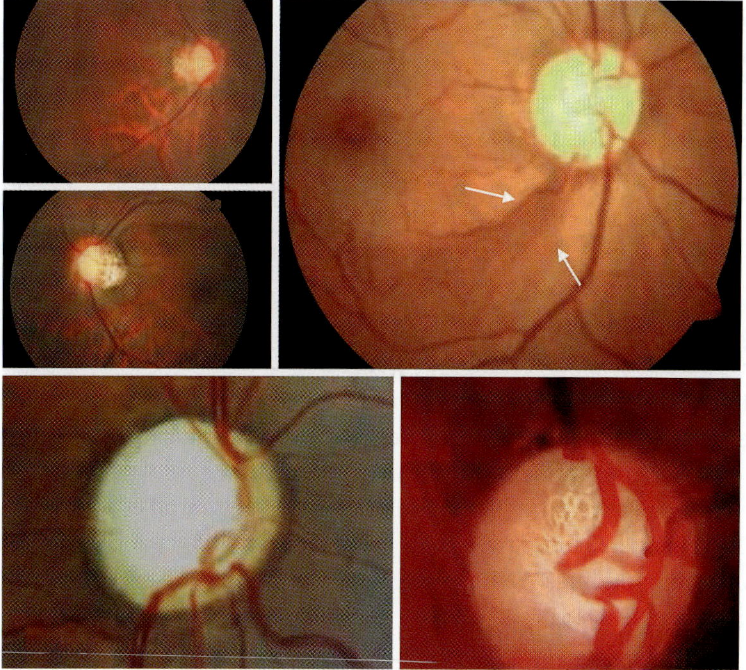

Fig. 4: Different stages of glaucoma.

To summarize, the journey of a glaucoma patient is not easy at all. At every stage, they look at you for hope. Be positive and help to spread positivity **(Fig. 4)**.

SUGGESTED READING

1. Lee PP. Outcomes and endpoints in glaucoma. J Glaucoma. 1996;5:295-7.

CHAPTER 14

Cases in Glaucoma

Rita Dhamankar, Roopali Nerlikar

CASE 1

A 64-year-old male presented for a routine eye checkup. History of (H/o) hypertension on treatment since 4 years. No other significant relevant history was noted. On examination, best corrected visual acuity (BCVA): 6/6, N6 OU. Intraocular pressure (IOP): 18 and 20 mm Hg. Central corneal thickness (CCT) 524 and 520 µm. Angles wide open to ciliary body band (CBB) in both eyes/all other findings WNL.

Did We Anything Different?

The fundus in the left eye showed a larger cup-to-disc (C/D) ratio as compared with the right eye. The inferior rim was thin, with a subtle retinal nerve fiber layer (RNFL) defect in the inferior temporal region. But the 24-2 Sita std showed almost no defect on perimetry. Just to confirm, we did the 24-2C Sita faster, which tests 10 additional central points and helps pick-up central defects faster. We also did the 10-2 to confirm our findings, and the 10-2 showed a definite defect. The optical coherence tomography (OCT) enhanced our belief. We had structure and function correlation. Newer testing modalities help early diagnosis **(Figs. 1 to 3)**.

Always try and do a structure-function correlation. If the RNFL defect was picked up on fundus examination, we should see if that can be correlated

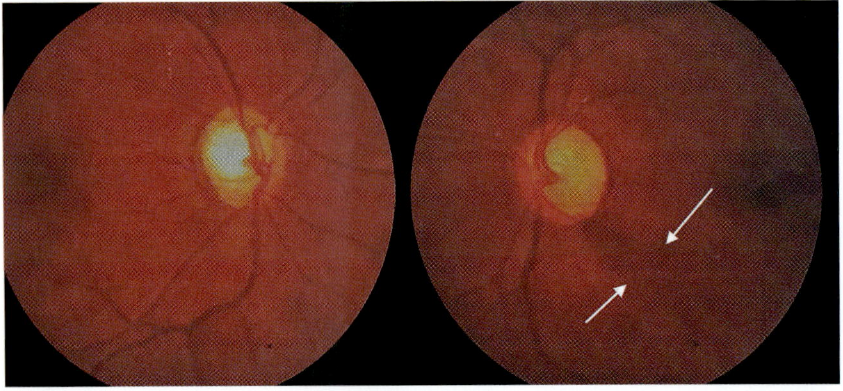

Fig. 1: Fundus both eyes.

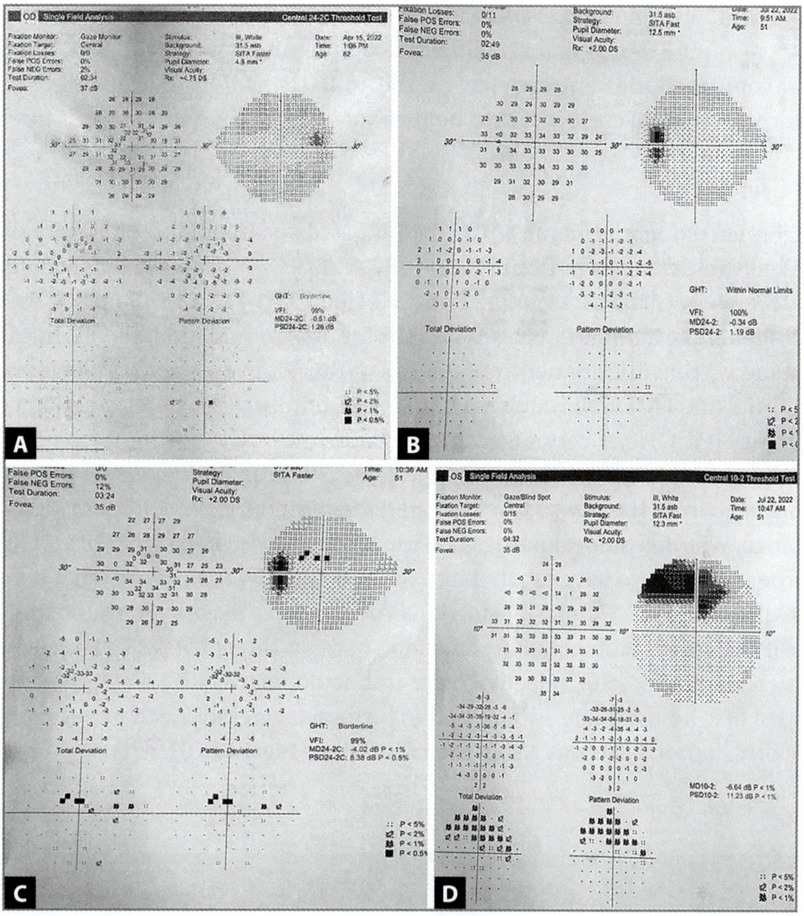

Figs. 2A to D: (A) 24-2C RE; (B) 24-2 SITA left eye; (C) 24-2C Sita Fast left eye; (D) 10-2 left eye.

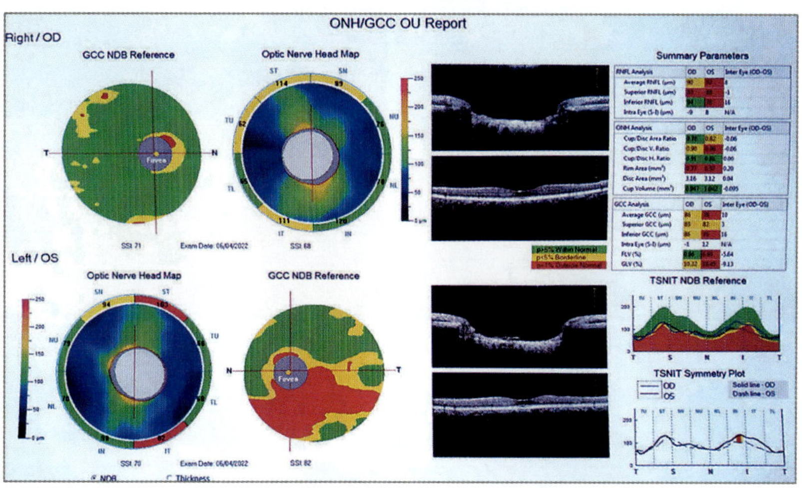

Fig. 3: Optical coherence tomography (OCT) both eyes.

with OCT, we not only got the same on OCT, but going one step ahead we were also able to detect a visual field defect on the newer 24-2C Sita Faster and confirmed the central defect on the 10-2. Using tests appropriately and interpreting them correctly, thus help us solve cases, if we are keen observers.

CASE 2

A 57-year-old female came with a h/o blurred vision off and on. There was no relevant history. On examination: BCVA 6/9/N6 OU. Early lens changes were seen in OU. IOP: 24 and 22 mm Hg and CCT: 484 and 490 µm. Rest of the slit lamp examination was WNL. On fundus examination, the RE fundus did show a thin inferior neuroretinal rim (NRR). Both eyes perimetry was still doubtful and OCT RNFL showed both RNFL thinning as well as ganglion cell complex (GCC) loss, very suggestive of glaucoma.

What would we label such a glaucoma? Was the finding on perimetry a learning curve? What next? We repeated the perimetry, we could not see any change. Was this preperimetric glaucoma? Patient also had high IOP and thin corneas. Could we have labeled him as an ocular hypertension? What about the disc changes? Should we start treatment/keep a close watch? Looking at the thin corneas with high IOP, I decided to treat. Target IOP was in the teens, which we got to, with selective laser trabeculoplasty (SLT). Later, he came with a disc hemorrhage and we had to be more aggressive with treatment, as the disc hemorrhage was a sign of progression **(Figs. 4 to 6)**.

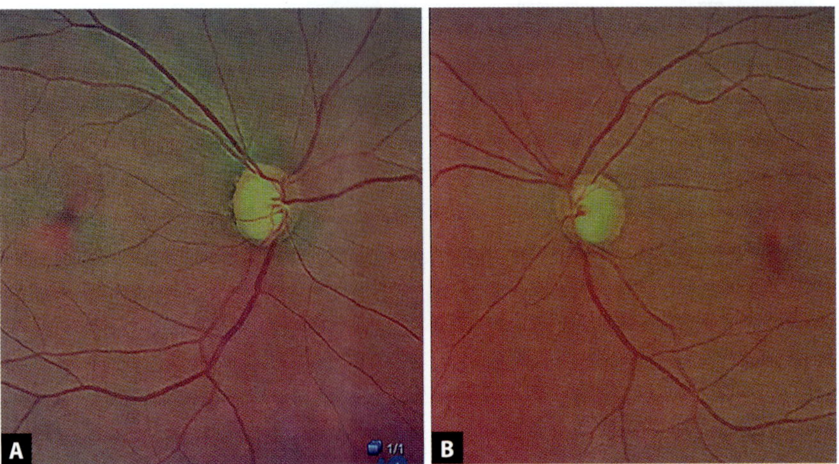

Figs. 4A and B: Fundus at presentation OD and (B) Fundus at presentation OS.

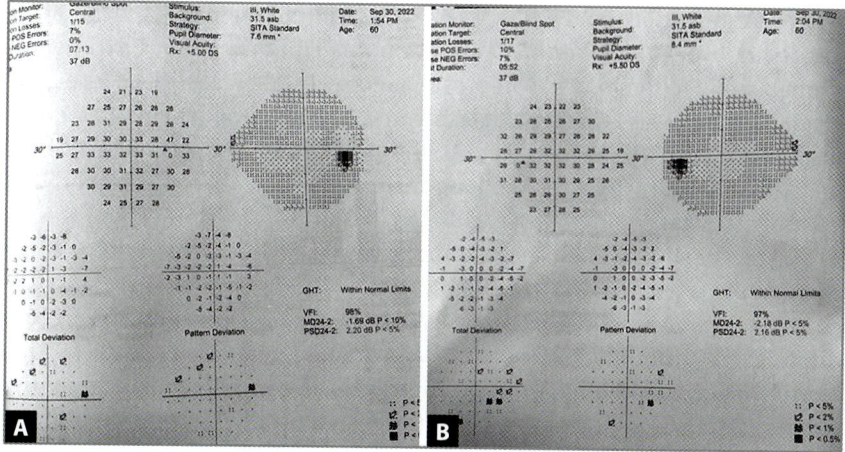

Figs. 5A and B: Perimetry 24-2 both eyes.

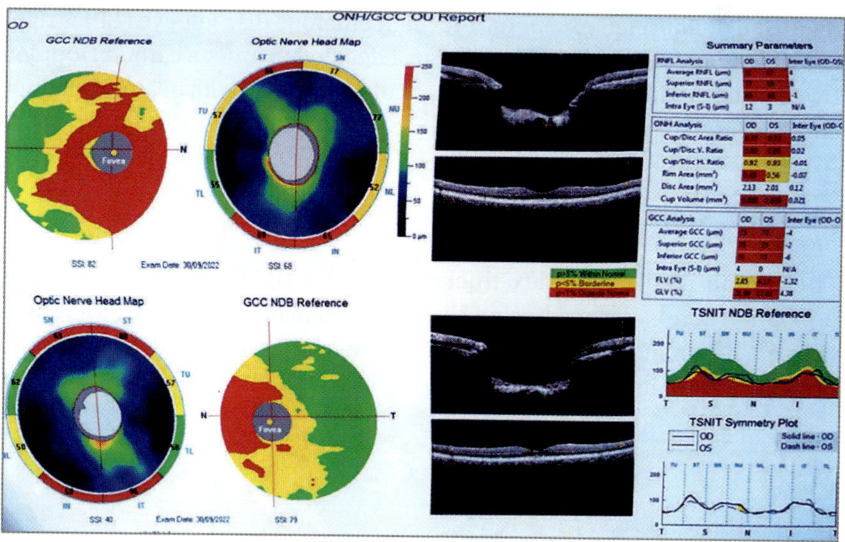

Fig. 6: Optical coherence tomography (OCT) BE.

CASE 3

A 74-year-old male patient presented with an acute loss of vision in the left eye. He was a known case of primary open-angle glaucoma (POAG) and was under treatment for the same for the last 12 years. Apparently stable. No h/o hypertension or diabetes. He had bilateral quiet pseudophakia.

On examination, his BCVA was 6/12, N12 in the right eye, and FC 1 foot in the left eye. On slit lamp examination, his conjunctiva was hyperemic, probably due to the long use of prostaglandin (PG) analogs. His cornea was clear. His pupil was reacting sluggishly in the right eye, but semidilated and fixed in the left eye. His IOPs were 12 mm Hg in both eyes with a CCT of 474 and 490 µm. This was a case of long-term POAG/?NTG, on treatment, well controlled, what could have been the cause for loss of vision? There was no h/o hypertension/diabetes. Could be a retinal detachment? Why was the right pupil sluggish?

Was it glaucoma progression? Why was the vision only in one eye diminished? From the history, there was no pain, redness, and just sudden loss of vision. Could it be a vitreous hemorrhage or a retinal detachment or some retinal pathology or some central visual problem? How should one proceed?

We had to have a look at the retina to rule out retinal pathologies.

Fundus seemed OK **(Figs. 7 and 8)**. There was no retinal vein occlusion, retina looked normal, except for the glaucomatous disc left eye (LE) > right eye (RE). Looking at his history and age, I decided to order a carotid Doppler. He came back with a report of bilateral ocular ischemia, with bilateral plaques and increased resistivity index.

B-mode Carotid Doppler

Right

The intima-media complex thickness in the right common carotid is 0.79 mm. There was a hyperechoic intraluminal plaque measuring 6.1 mm in length, 1.1 mm in thickness seen on the posterior wall of the distal common carotid artery at its bifurcation.

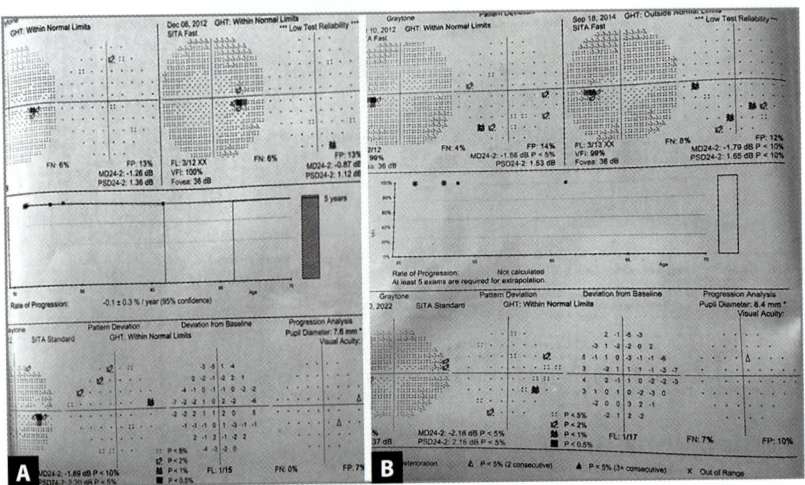

Figs. 7A and B: Glaucoma progression analysis on perimetry both eyes.

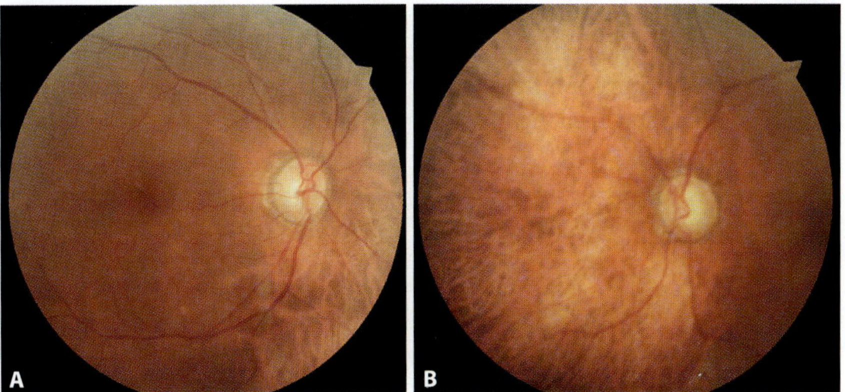

Figs. 8A and B: Fundus examination of both the (A) Right and (B) Left.

Left

The intima-media complex thickness in the left common carotid was 0.73 mm. There is a hyperechoic intraluminal plaque measuring 6.3 mm in length, 1.8 mm in thickness, seen on the posterior wall of the distal common carotid artery at its bifurcation.

Resistivity index and the pulsatility index were high in the ophthalmic arteries, posterior ciliary arteries, and the central retinal arteries.

Right central retinal vein showed low flow velocities.

Plaque (grade 4) was noted in the common carotid arteries at its bifurcation. Thickened intima was noted in the common carotid arteries. *Suggestive of atherosclerotic changes.*

Ocular color and spectral Doppler studies are suggestive of ocular ischemic syndrome, left is more severe than the right. Low velocity flow in the left central retinal artery is suggestive of occlusion.

What next? A cardiologist's opinion was sought. He has been put on statins. He has recovered his vision partially which improved to 6/9, N6 and 6/24, and N8. Continued the same treatment and was on a regular monitoring. He has come in the last year with three attacks of transient ischemic attacks lasting for a few hours and getting back to previous vision. It is important for us to remember that a patient with long-standing well-controlled glaucoma could also have other systemic comorbidities contributing to reduction in vision. Commonly, hypertension, atherosclerosis, and diabetes of long-standing contribute to poor vision thus. We cannot forget neurological causes like multiple sclerosis presenting with optic neuritis either.

CASE 4

A 43-year-old female comes with a h/o diminished vision in the right eye since a few years. She has no h/o injury, ocular surgery, steroid use, hypertension, diabetes, and family h/o glaucoma. Her diminished vision is sometimes associated with a headache, but there are no aggravating/alleviating factors.

She has seen many ophthalmologists in the past who have given her some eyedrops, which she used inconsistently, with no relief.

On examination:

OD	*OS*
BCVA: HM	6/6/N6
GAT: 64 mm Hg	16 mm Hg
Cornea: WNL	WNL
AC: Irregular	WNL
Peripheral anterior synechiae (PAS) temporally	
IRIS: Dark small nodules	WNL
Pupil: Ectropion uvea	Round reacting briskly to light
Corectopia	
Lens: Clear	Clear
Fundus: Glaucomatous	WNL
Optic neuropathy	

Diagnosis was very clear. It is a variant of the iridocorneal endothelial (ICE) syndrome, namely Cogan-Reese syndrome, which is a very rare disorder that predominantly affects females in the middle adult years. Family history usually shows no other affected family members.

Major characteristics of Cogan-Reese syndrome include:

- Matted or smudged appearance to the surface of the iris (nevus)
- Yellow or brown lumps or nodules on the iris (nodular iris nevi)
- Attachment of portions of the iris to the cornea (peripheral anterior synechiae)
- Increased pressure in the eye (glaucoma).

The matted appearance of the iris and development of nodules on the iris distinguish Cogan-Reese syndrome from the other iridocorneal endothelial syndromes.

Other features of Cogan-Reese syndrome may include:

- Swelling of the cornea (corneal edema)
- Abnormalities in the cells lining the cornea (corneal endothelium).

These changes may be responsible for the glaucoma that is characteristic of this disorder. People who develop glaucoma may also develop:

- Eye pain or headache if they have a severe increase in IOP due to secondary glaucoma.

- Blurred vision
- A decrease in vision sharpness or severe vision loss
- Changes in the appearance of the iris, where the edge of the pupil may turn outward (ectropion uveae) and/or a transparent membrane may appear across the surface of the iris.

Cogan-Reese syndrome, like other ICE syndromes, causes significant changes in both the structure and function of the eye. In Cogan-Reese syndrome, the mechanism of glaucoma is believed to be related to a cellular membrane secreted by the abnormal endothelial cells. This membrane covers the trabecular meshwork of the drainage angle, thereby obstructing aqueous outflow facility and elevating IOP, leading to glaucoma.

Specular microscopy examines the cornea's endothelial tissue to assess its health. It shows the typical ICE cells, with loss of endothelial cells and change in morphology **(Figs. 9 to 11)**.

Typically, the treatment for glaucoma is to keep the IOP low and try to preserve vision. This can be achieved by medications, but better still surgically, typically trabeculectomies do not do so well. Tubes is the surgery of choice. The cornea is also known to decompensate over a period of time, when doing a Descemet's stripping automated endothelial keratoplasty (DSAEK) is the only way out.

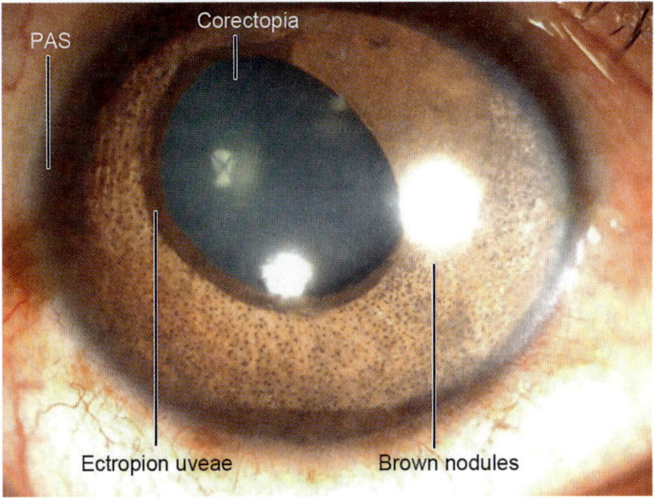

Fig. 9: Slit lamp examination of the RE, which depicts a correctopia semidialted with ectropion pupillae, Brown nodules on the iris and Peripheral anterior synechiae. (PAS: peripheral anterior synechiae)

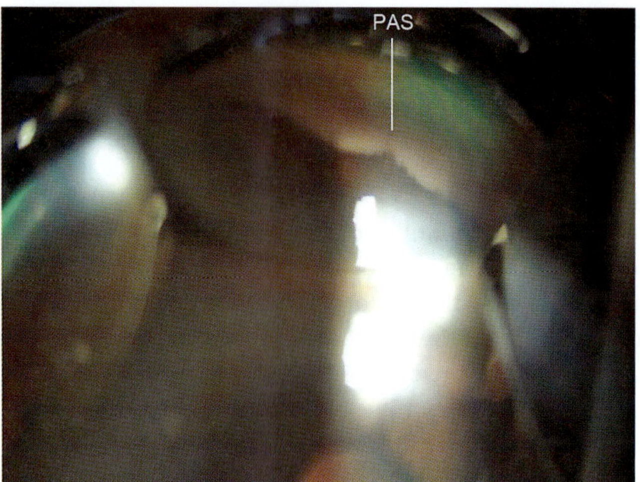

Fig. 10: PAS: Peripheral anterior synechiae.

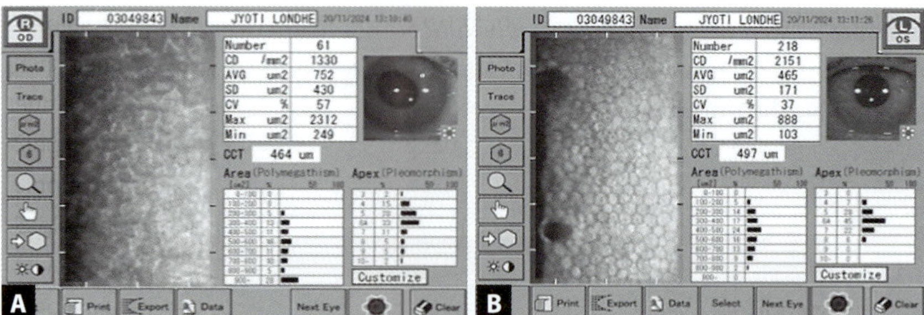

Figs. 11A and B: (A) Iridocorneal endothelial (ICE) cells; (B) Specular microscopy of the corneal endothelium.

CASE 5

A 26-year-old male patient came with a h/o juvenile-onset open-angle glaucoma (JOAG) diagnosed elsewhere, on MMT for the last year, but with pressures not responding. Family h/o glaucoma in two siblings and one paternal aunt. Aunt gave a h/o going blind in one eye, due to glaucoma by the age of 40 years. No other relevant history noted. On examination, patient's BCVA was 6/6, N6 and 6/9, and N8, respectively. His IOPs were 24 and 28 mm Hg, with CCT of 520 and 512 μm, respectively. He had long dark eyelashes in both eyes, with a very hyperemic conjunctiva.

OU, and a lusterless cornea in OU. Schirmer's confirmed the diagnosis of dry eye with Schirmer's reading of 2 mm at the end of 5 minutes. His anterior chambers (ACs) were normal and angles on gonioscopy were open till the ciliary band body. Iris was normal in pattern; pupils were round and reacting briskly to light. Lenses were clear in both the eyes. The fundus looked as shown in **Figures 12A and B.**

The fundus **Figures 13A and B** show us pretty advanced damage to the optic nerve head LE > RE, as the upper and lower rims in the right eye can still be seen. The perimetry 24-2 in the RE shows an inferior hemifield defect with a superior nasal defect. With a visual field index (VFI) of 66% and a mean deviation (MD) of –16.88 dB. The left eye perimetry shows a generalized defect with nothing showing on the pattern standard deviation, which tells you that the MD must be >20 dB due to advanced disease. Here, the VFI is

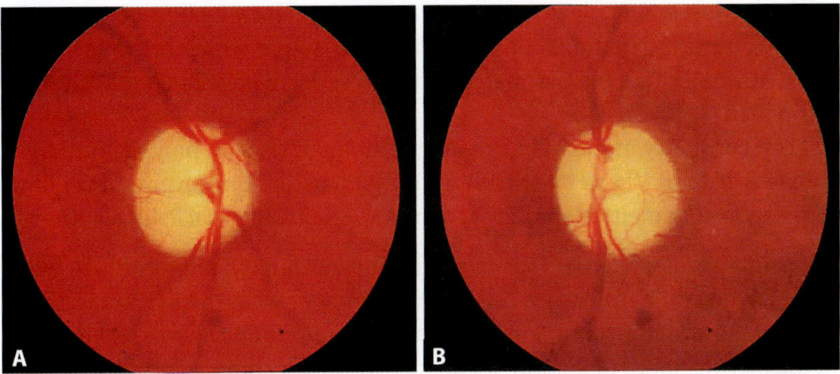

Figs. 12A and B: Advanced glaucomatous optic atrophy with pallor in both eyes and large cups with a very thin NRR.

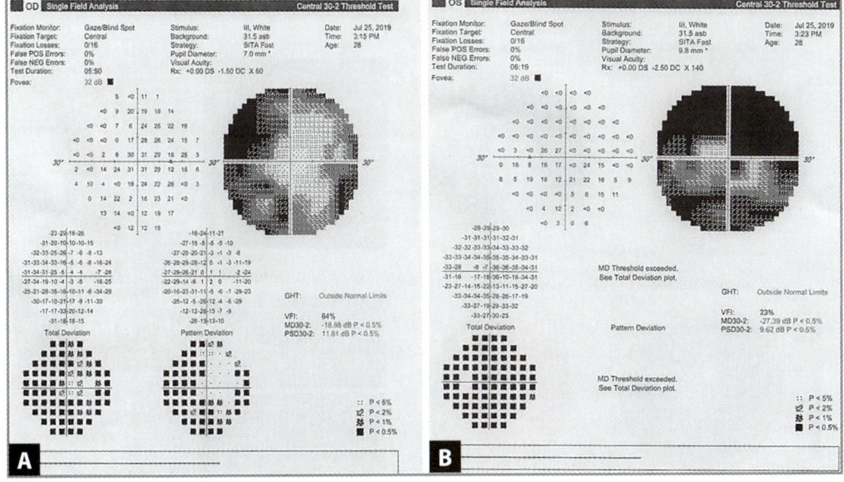

Figs. 13A and B: (A) Perimetry 24-2 OD and (B) Perimetry 24-2 OS.

23% with a MD of –27.88 dB, hence, there is no pattern standard deviation shown. Diagnosis of advanced JOAG, LE > RE was made. Despite having such an advanced disease, the vision was still pretty good, and that was because on the gray scale you can see that the central visual field is well maintained. *Never forget to look at the fundus in every eye, despite vision being recorded to be near normal.* At this point, I decided to operate on both the eyes, as patient was very young, had advanced glaucoma, with a bad family history, and IOPs still not on target, which should have been episcleral venous pressure.

For the sake of completion, also got an OCT done, which showed marked thinning of RNFL in both eyes with an equally severe loss of GCC.

Proceeded as per plan, it was successful in getting the IOPs down to 18 mm Hg in the RE and 14 mm Hg in the left eye, after watching the IOP at 12 weeks post-trabeculectomy with mitomycin C (MMC) in BE, started the patient on a prostaglandin analog in the RE. Together with lubricants in both eyes. We shall share his perimetry on follow-up. We have been following up this patient regularly.

The perimetry in the right eye on granulomatosis with polyangiitis (GPA) shows a drop in VFI to start with and then a stable improvement till date. Whereas the perimetry in the left eye shows a very stable visual fields all through.

Points to be noted: Remember to always look at the dilated fundus in every patient who comes to you for refraction, no matter what their vision is.

Doing a structure-function correlation is important. Do not treat the RED in the investigation, make sure it concurs with your clinical findings.

Always document your findings, a perimetry with MD > –20 dB will never show you a pattern standard deviation, go ahead and do a 10-2 to look for the central vision. Ensure that you start with a new baseline post any intervention.

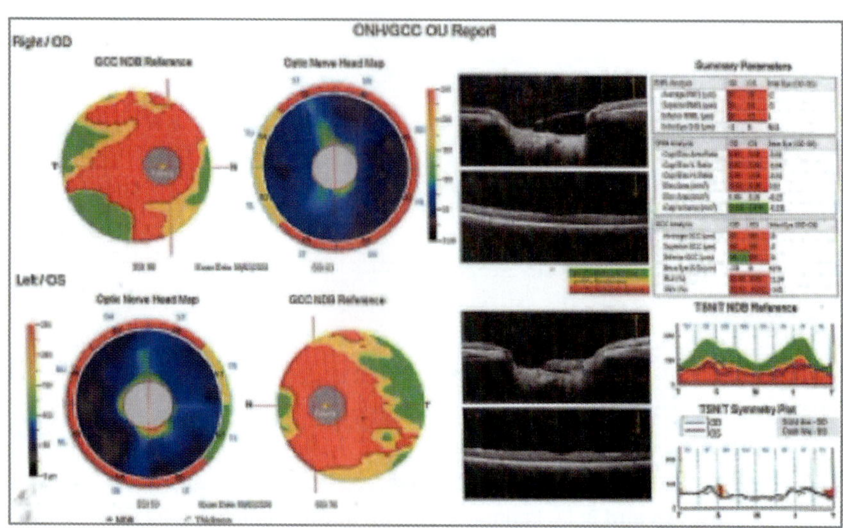

Fig. 14: Optical coherence tomography (OCT) glaucoma OU.

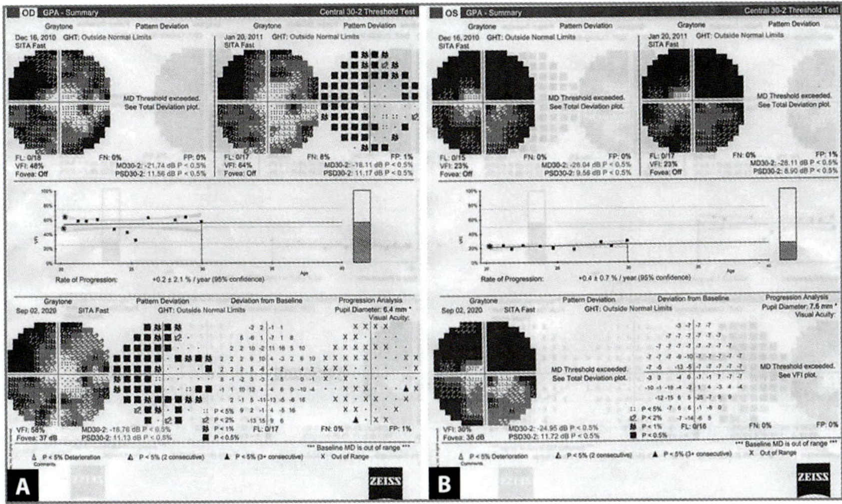

Figs. 15A and B: Glaucoma progression analysis OU. (A) Right eye; (B) Left eye.

In advanced glaucomas, OCT cannot be used to look for progression, you have to take recourse to perimetry, as that will give you important data. Remember the OCT values of RNFL only vary between 80 and 40 µm in glaucoma. There is always a floor effect seen below 30–40 µm, hence, further thinning cannot be documented on an OCT.

Never lose hope, even in advanced cases, do all you can to maintain vision for your patient. See how well the patient's vision has been preserved for the last 8 years, just by a regular follow-up, after a bold decision to intervene surgically **(Figs. 14 and 15)**.

CASE 6

A 34-year-old female patient presented with complaining of (c/o) headaches occasional with marked photophobia. She was seen by numerous ophthalmologists, neurologists, and even a psychiatrist for the last 2 years. All her imaging studies were normal. Her counseling sessions had not helped. She was an intellect, who had to give up her managerial position in an MNC abroad as she was unable to perform.

On examination, her BCVA was 6/6, N6 in OU. External examination was within normal limits. Her IOP were 12 and 18 mm Hg. Her CCT was 522 and 528 µm. Her fundus shown in **Figure 16**.

There seemed to be disc asymmetry, with the left eye definitely showing a larger cup with no inferior rim, a RNFL defect in the inferotemporal region. The fundus in the right eye also showed a C/D ratio of 0.65 with no other changes.

Her perimetry and OCT were WNL. This did not get me very far. I did a diurnal variation to confirm normal tension glaucoma and her highest with

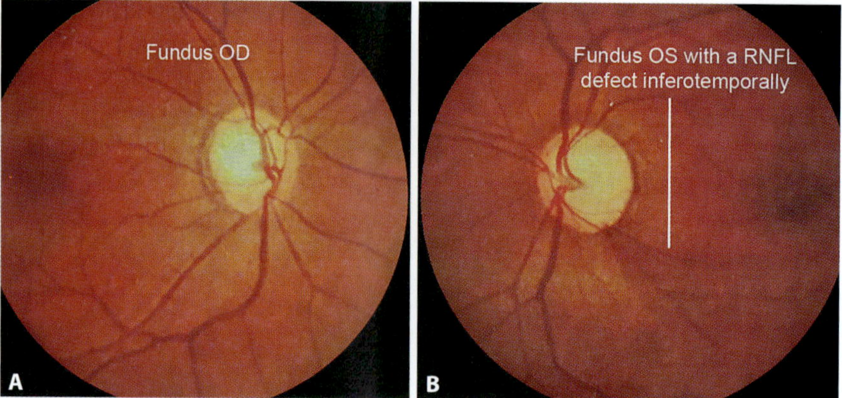

Figs. 16A and B: (A): Fundus OD and (B) Fundus OS with a retinal nerve fiber layer (RNFL) defect inferotemporally.

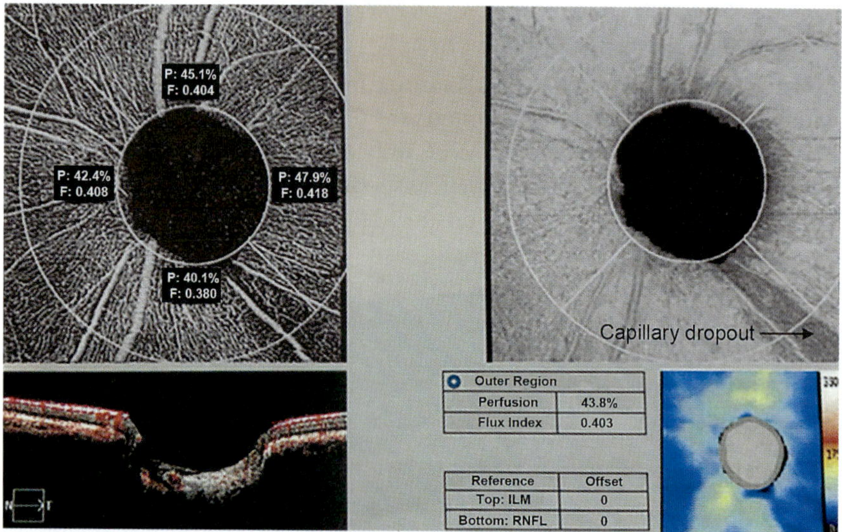

Fig. 17: Optical coherence tomography angiography (OCTA) OS.

a variation of 5 mm through 24 hours. I was still lost. By which time optical coherence tomography angiography (OCTA) had become available for clinical use **(Fig. 17)**.

So, I decided to get an OCTA done. The capillary dropout in the left eye is seen very clearly. This tells you that there is a beginning of pathology in the RNFL in that area. Could I label this as preperimetric glaucoma? NO, there were no RNFL changes or GCC loss seen on OCT. But remember the *glaucoma continuum* **(Fig. 18)**.

We are somewhere close to the arrow in the continuum. What next? She definitely was a normal tension glaucoma with proven vascular dropout.

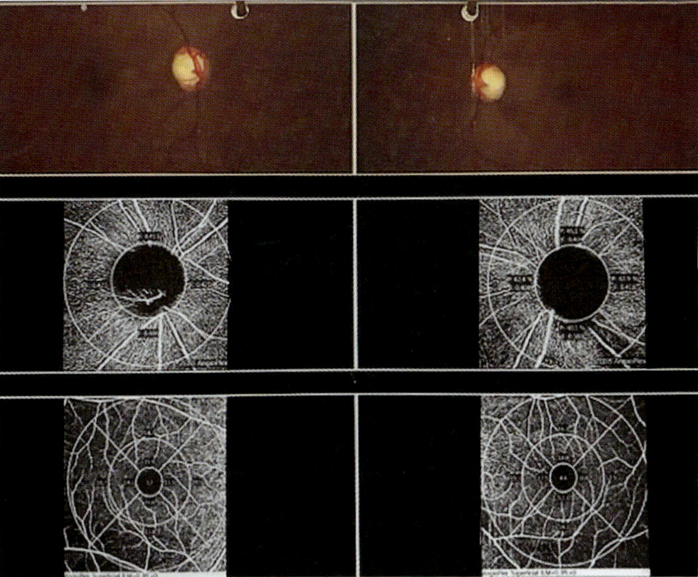

Fig. 18: Optical coherence tomography angiography (OCTA) OU.

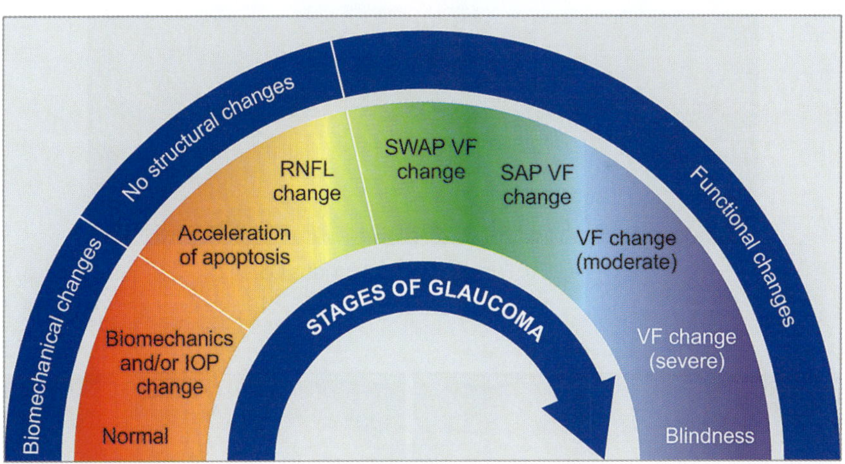

Fig. 19: CONTINUUM of Glaucoma.

She was young, she needed to preserve her eyesight. I decided to treat her as NTG. For the last 4 years, she has been almost steady. Last month her OCT for the first time showed an RNFL thinning in the inferior temporal quadrant of the LE. Perimetry is WNL. Vision continues to remain stable. She has started working comfortably. Rehabilitated a young lady with the use of advanced technology **(Fig. 19)**.

CASE 7

A 64-year-old female came for a second opinion for glaucoma, with no ocular complaint. She was a hypertensive, with a h/o stroke in the past on treatment.

History of diabetes mellitus (DM) on treatment. No family history of (f/h/o) glaucoma. No h/o of ocular trauma/surgery in the past. She was not on any steroids, topically/systemically. She did have h/o occasional headaches and no other associated symptoms.

BCVA: 6/6, N6 OU. AC was shallow with a sine wave sign. OU pupil round reacting briskly OU lens showed early NS OU. GAT: 28 and 32 mm Hg. CCT: 512 and 516 μm **(Figs. 20 and 21)**.

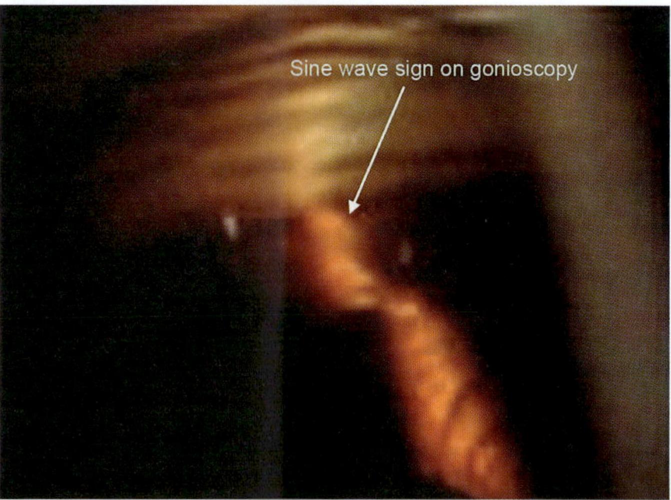

Fig. 20: Fundus OD and fundus OS.

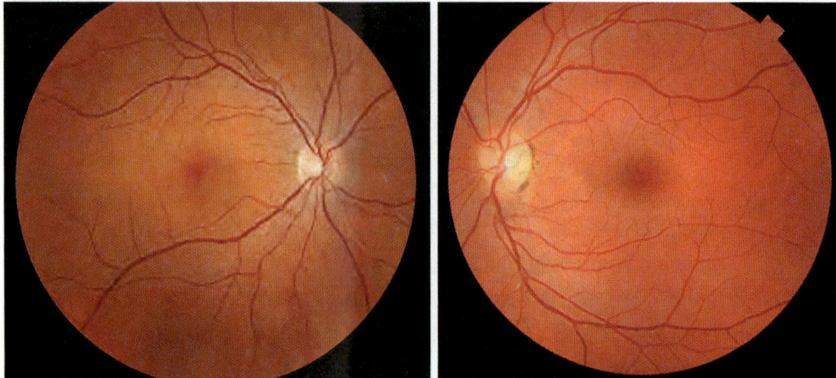

Fig. 21: Fundus pictures in the RE and LE.

Investigations

- Which ones? Perimetry. Looking at the fundus do you expect any abnormalities?
- OCT? Can you foresee any structural defects?
- Diagnosis of primary angle closure OU with a plateau iris configuration, with high intraocular pressures was made.
- *Risk factors:* Systemic hypertension with a h/o stroke DM on treatment. Early cataracts with lens thickness of 5.02 and 5.08.
- Did a peripheral iridotomy. Will cataract extraction open the angles and relieve the closure? (EAGLE STUDY) We had to bring the IOP down. Was not confident about (ALPI) iridoplasty. With 3 AGM's IOPs remained at 22 mm Hg. Lots of redness and unhappy patient. Opted to do a cataract extraction with IOL with trabeculectomy with MMC. Both eyes did very well, IOP came down to the mid-teens with a diffuse bleb.
- Three months later, patient came back with a sudden loss of vision in the left eye. What could have gone wrong? Cause for sudden loss of vision post-trabeculectomy? Infection/injury/vascular accident/vitreous hemorrhage/retinal detachment. The vision in the LE had come down to FC 1 ft. IOP was 4 mm Hg. The bleb was diffuse. Seidel's test was negative. The cornea showed some haze. AC was very shallow. Early choroidals seen. With such a soft eye, gonioscopy was difficult to do. No h/o injury to the eye for a cyclodialysis cleft. Siedel's test and forced Seidel's test was negative. Formed AC on the table with Healon GV. Did a gonioscopy to look for a cleft. Did not see one. Patched the patient after adding a bandage contact lens (BCL). Started systemic steroids and topical atropine. 4 days later came back again with similar complaints **(Fig. 22)**.

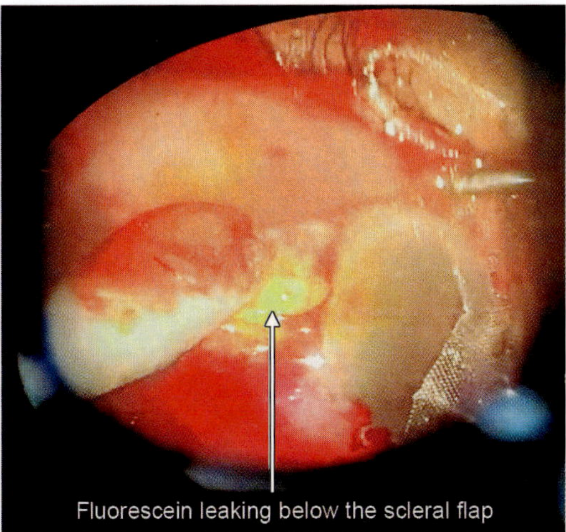

Fig. 22: Diagnoses a leak in the wound.

- Obviously, our diagnosis of a leak was probably right, from where? All tests were nonconclusive. I decided to open up the bleb to see if the scleral flap sutures were loose. Had to cut two sutures. One had been released earlier. After dissecting the superficial flap. To my surprise I found a small leak beneath the superficial flap on the scleral bed. It did not look a scleral melt. Scleral fistula? We could see fluorescein run along with the leak. We had to close the fistula. A partial scleral graft was glued onto the defect, conjunctival sutured, the AC formed on the table.

Postsurgery, patient had a well-formed AC, choroidals regressed, and the vision came back to 6/9, N6, with IOP of 14 mm Hg. Continues to do well.

Remember, the goal is do no harm, but not leave the patient to fend for himself. If it means opening up to search for the problem, be bold, identify the problem. and treat it. If you are not confident, please refer it to someone who can, but save the patient's eye.

CASE 8

Sturge-Weber syndrome (SWS) case of secondary glaucoma **(Fig. 23)**.

A 24-year-old female came for a second opinion after being diagnosed to have been operated for trabeculectomy with uncontrolled pressures.

On examination, she had a *port wine stain on the right side of her face, involving the lids of the right eye, going onto the forehead.*

She did have a h/o seizures for which she was on treatment.

She had BCVA: 6/6, N6 in both eyes. Her IOP: 28 and16 mm Hg. Her CCT was 512 and 506 µm, respectively. She had a flat diffuse bleb in the right eye, with a clear cornea, deep AC, and a clear lens. Her fundus *did not show a choroidal hemangioma,* the disc was normal with a C/D ratio of 0.8 with thin superior and inferior rims. Her LE was WNL.

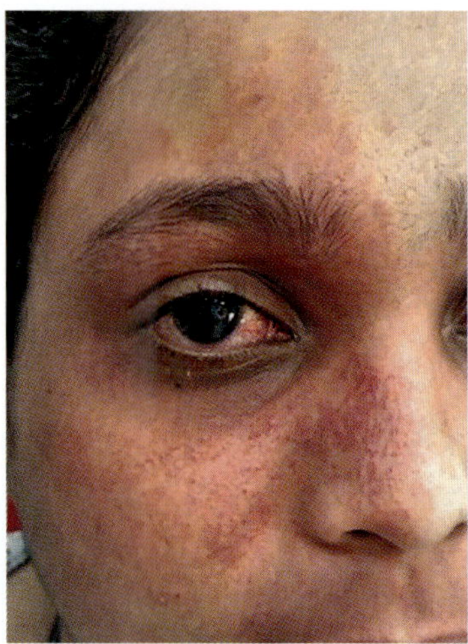

Fig. 23: Face typically seen in Sturge Weber's Syndrome.

A diagnosis of a secondary glaucoma due to SWS status post-trabeculectomy with uncontrolled pressures was made in the right eye with a normal left eye. Her pressures needed to be lowered. Tried with MMT for a few months, but saw not much lowering. Patient *had tortuous episcleral veins*, deep red eyes with a lot of discomfort. Opted to do an Ahmed glaucoma valve and succeeded in bringing the IOP down to 12 mm Hg in 6 months. 3 years later, stays at 12 mm Hg with one AGM.

Her perimetry findings have always posed a problem as she had a picture showing a homonymous hemianopia.

Cause for homonymous hemianopia: Homonymous hemianopia is a visual field defect involving either the two right or the two left halves of the visual fields of both eyes. It is caused by lesions of the retro chiasmal visual pathways, i.e., lesions of the optic tract, the lateral geniculate nucleus, the optic radiations, and the cerebral visual (occipital) cortex **(Figs. 24A and B)**.

Any type of intracranial lesion in the appropriate location can cause a homonymous hemianopia; however, vascular causes (cerebral infarction and intracranial hemorrhage) are the most frequent in adults, ranging from 42 to 89%, followed by brain tumors, trauma, surgical interventions, and other central nervous system diseases. In children, neoplasms are the most common cause of homonymous hemianopia (39%), followed by cerebrovascular disease (25%), and trauma (19%). Uncommon causes of homonymous hemianopia include multiple sclerosis, infections (encephalitis and abscess), degenerative dementia (posterior cortical atrophy), Creutzfeldt-Jakob disease, adrenoleukodystrophy, seizures, and severe hyperglycemia. Got an

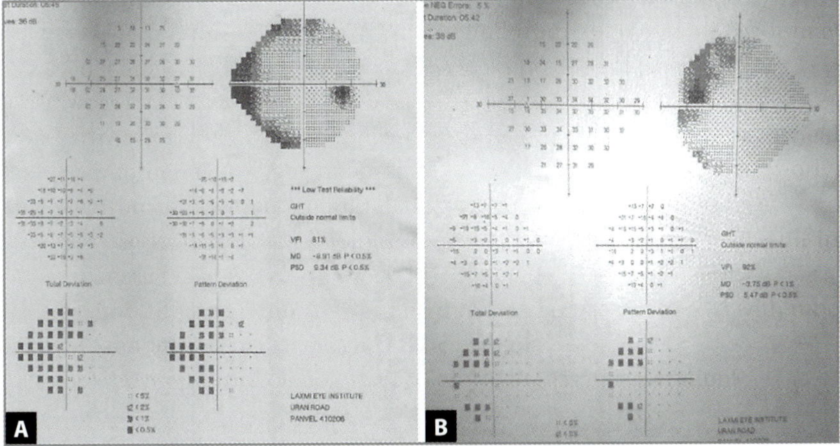

Figs. 24A and B: (A) Perimetry od showing a vertical hemianopia nasally; (B) Perimetry os showing a vertical hemianopia temporally.

MRI done, which was normal. Attributed this to seizures that the patient had due to SWS.

Cause for secondary glaucoma: The two main mechanisms of glaucoma in SWS are malformation of the AC angle and an elevated episcleral venous pressure. Our patient had a normal AC and we had to attribute the cause to elevated episcleral venous pressure, therefore, the appearance of dilated episcleral veins seen in the right eye.

Points to note: Any unilateral glaucoma has to be looked into differently for a specific cause.

Perimetry has to be interpreted rationally.

CASE 9

Fast progression of angle-closure glaucoma **(Fig. 25)**.

A 48-year-old male patient came to us for glaucoma evaluation as he had positive f/h/o glaucoma.

On examination, BCVA in both eyes was 6/9, N6. IOP in right and left eye was 24 and 20 mm Hg. Anterior segment examination showed peripherally shallow ACs with patent peripheral iridotomies. Retinal examination revealed C/D ratio 0.85 bipolar thinning in the right eye and 0.6 in the left eye, respectively. Perimetry showed inferior arcuate scotoma in right eye and left eye was within normal limits with pachymetry of 470 and 475 μm right and left eye, respectively **(Fig. 26)**.

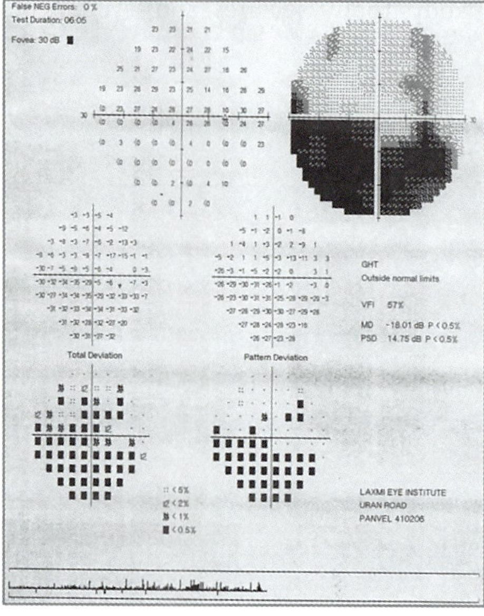

Fig. 25: Perimetry OD.

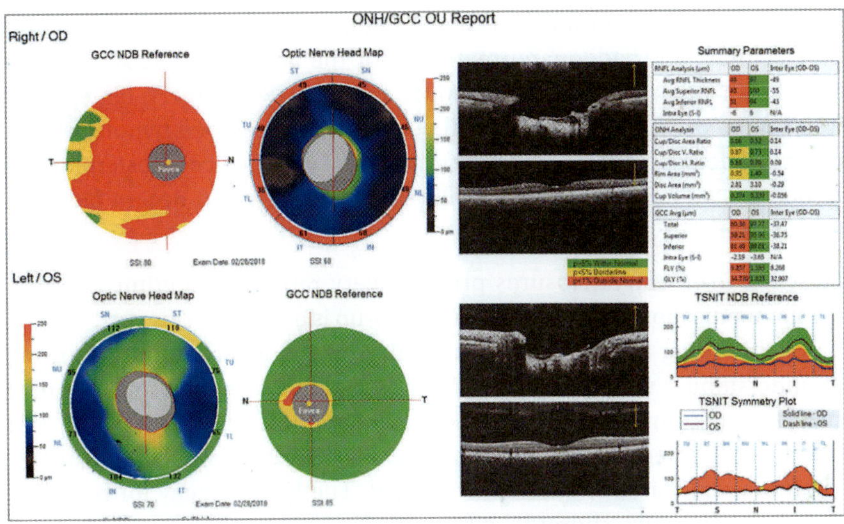

Fig. 26: Optical coherence tomography (OCT) glaucoma OU.

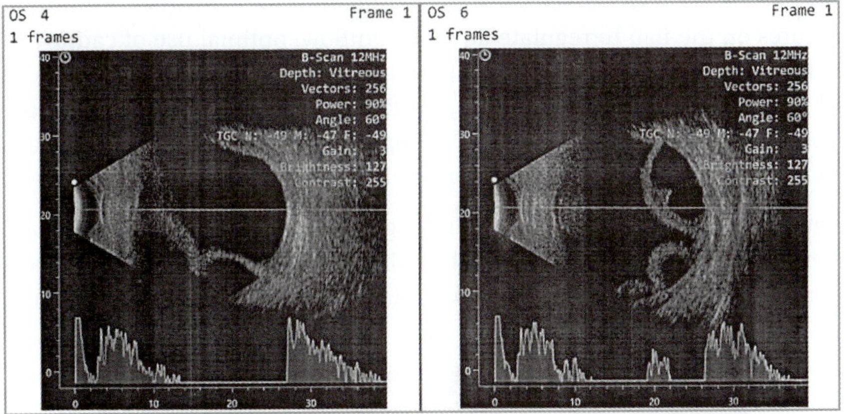

Fig. 27: B-scan OS showing choroidal detachment.

Patient was started on a combination of bimatoprost and β-blocker eye drop in both eyes which reduced his IOP in left eye to 12 mm Hg but right eye IOP to 22 mm Hg. Added a dorzolamide after adequate trial of above combination in the right eye. IOP reduced to 18 mm Hg. OCT in right eye suggestive of gross loss of GCC and left eye was within normal limits **(Fig. 27)**. Diagnosis of advanced primary angle closure glaucoma (PACG) was made in RE and target IOP was changed to episcleral venous pressure.

Hence, patient underwent trabeculectomy with MMC in right eye, surgery was uneventful, and IOP came down to 12 mm Hg. Postoperatively he was finally asked to continue medications only in the left eye. On one successive follow-up, he came back with an acute angle closure in his left eye with his

IOP in left eye at 50 mm Hg, and pain, redness, despite the patent PI and medications. After adequate treatment for the acute angle closure, went ahead with a trabeculectomy with MMC in the LE. Postsurgery, left eye IOP was 8 mm Hg. In successive follow-ups, patient developed hypotony with choroidal detachment for which he was treated with oral corticosteroids. He responded well to steroids and finally settled down with a decent bleb and IOP of 14 mm Hg.

Lessons learnt: Angle closures progress very rapidly, sometimes despite regular medications. So, a very close follow-up is a must.

Shepherding a bleb, post a trabeculectomy is a very important thing to understand. Even in the best of hands, a trabeculectomy may not be a success every time immediately postoperative. It is the shepherding that helps you to intervene at the right time, like this patient with choroidals. There was no leak, the sutures were tight. The best strategy for handling acute intraoperative choroidal effusions is to prevent them by minimizing hypotony and inflammation intraoperatively and postoperatively **(Fig. 28)**.

During surgery: Good scleral flap architecture and thickness, multiple sutures on the flap to regulate aqueous outflow, optimal use of cautery to achieve hemostasis but no scarring or thinning of the sclera, judicious use of antimetabolites, placement of anterior sclerotomy to avoid the ciliary body, and meticulous closure of the conjunctiva are all important measures to minimize intraoperative bleeding and hypotony during glaucoma surgery.

Drainage devices: For glaucoma drainage devices, one may opt for valved devices. For nonvalved devices, the tube should be ligated, or two-stage surgery may be performed to allow formation of a fibrous capsule around

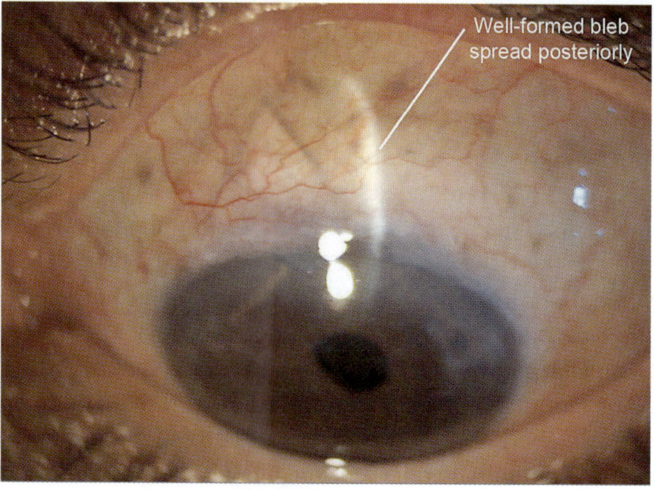

Fig. 28: Well-formed bleb spread posteriorly.

the plate to avoid excessive filtration in the early postoperative period, minimizing hypotony and its related sequelae.

High-risk patients: Prophylactic sclerotomies at the time of glaucoma filtration surgery may be helpful in high-risk cases with known susceptibility to choroidal effusions, such as patients with prior postoperative choroidal effusions, nanophthalmos, or SWS.

Postoperative care: Topical and systemic aqueous suppressants should be discontinued, and early laser suture lysis should be avoided.

Conclusion

Choroidal effusions may result from various etiologies but are most commonly encountered after glaucoma surgery, especially in the setting of hypotony, inflammation, or both. Meticulous surgical steps and preventive measures may help to reduce the risk of choroidal effusions. While most choroidal effusions resolve spontaneously, surgical drainage may be necessary in some cases to restore normal anatomy and visual function.

CASE 10

Masquerades

A 24-year-old male patient came to us for a second opinion as he had been diagnosed elsewhere as glaucoma and was started on three medications for the same. His complain was diminished vision in the right eye which was noticed at an eye examination done for a job. There was no other notable contributable cause to his glaucoma **(Figs. 29A and B)**.

On examination, his BCVA was 6/18 in the RE and 6/6, in the left eye. His AC was normal in BE with a clear lens. IOP was 18 mm Hg in both eyes. He had not started any medications. On fundus examination, this is what we saw.

What is your diagnosis? You would want to call this unilateral glaucoma affecting the RE?

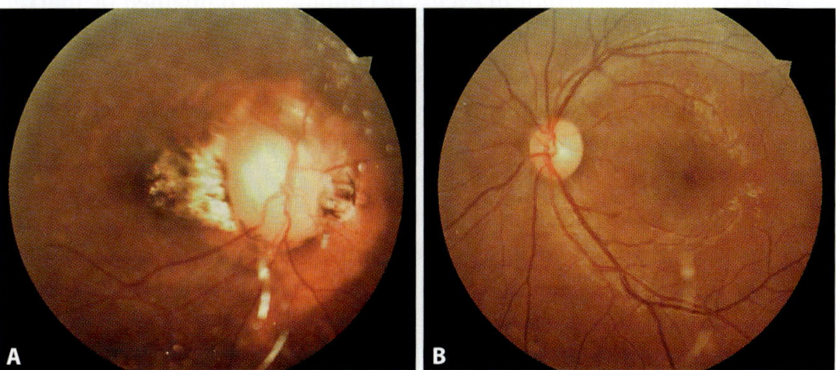

Figs. 29A and B: (A) Fundus OD (B) Fundus OS.

Stretch your imagination and see if the right disc looks glaucomatous? There is a marked difference in both the discs. Look at the size of the discs. Look at the margin of the discs? To my mind, this is a disc coloboma.

Many conditions can mimic glaucoma. They include:

- Compressive or infiltrative lesions of the optic nerve, previous ischemic optic neuropathy (both arteritic and nonarteritic)
- Congenital and hereditary optic neuropathies
- Post-traumatic optic neuropathy
- Inflammatory and demyelinating optic neuritis
- High myopia
- Most cases in the compressive category—intracranial space-occupying lesions (ICSOLs) that cause optic nerve or chiasmal compression will be: pituitary adenomas, craniopharyngiomas, suprasellar aneurysms or meningiomas. Many such tumors will present in patients who are younger than the average glaucoma patient. Patients with compressive injury may show visual fields resembling glaucoma, with arcuate or nerve fiber bundle loss and shallow optic disc cupping. *The optic nerve pallor is in excess of cupping, particularly of the temporal rim. A vertical step in the visual field* should also alert the clinician of possible compression or infiltration, as should *a cecocentral scotoma or decreased acuity.*
- Previous ischemic optic neuropathy may present with nerve fiber bundle field loss if seen after the disc swelling resolves. Arteritic ischemic optic neuropathy may result in cupping resembling glaucoma, from a loss of disc substance produced by profound ischemia diseases such as autosomal dominant optic atrophy, papillorenal syndrome, *optic nerve head pits and colobomas,* superior segmental optic nerve hypoplasia, and Leber's hereditary optic neuropathy can all mimic glaucoma. A careful history and the duration and/or progression of the clinical findings are helpful clues in establishing the correct diagnosis.
- Marked neural rim pallor in excess of cupping, accompanied by marked focal arterial narrowing near the disc, is common in anterior ischemic optic neuropathy (AION). The patient may give a h/o acute loss of vision with headache, jaw claudication, weight loss, anorexia, and fever.

  In nonarteritic ischemic optic neuropathy the contralateral disc may have a small cup; the involved eye may have altitudinal pallor without cupping, but with retinal arterial narrowing.
- Symmetrical scalloped blurred margins 360°, lumpy bumpy central elevation due to a small disc focal glossy nerve fiber layer (NFL), absent cup, and venous pulsations are seen in an optic nerve drusen.

  It is therefore very important to distinguish a true glaucoma from its masquerade. I have given **Figures 30A to I** of various masquerades.

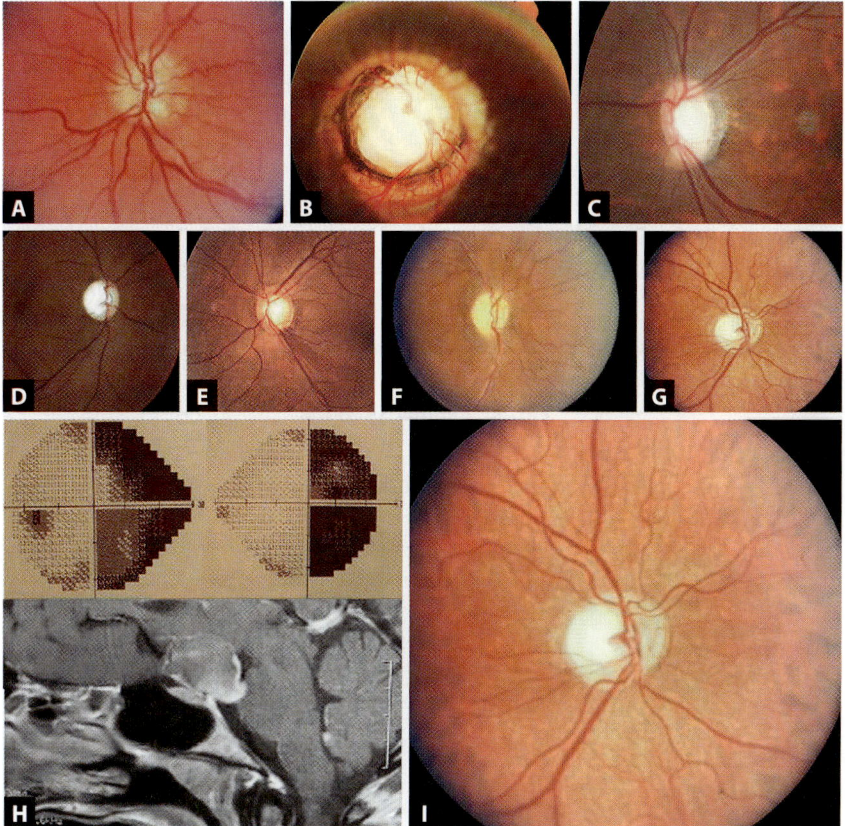

Figs. 30A to I: Various glaucoma masqueraders.

Now that I have described so many of them above, you can look at the **Figures 30A to I** and see how many you can identify. There are some common ones, such as a compressive lesion, an AION, myopia, and a morning glory syndrome.

CASE 11

Watchdog Perimetry. When to ask for a 10-2 (Fig. 31)?

A 53-year-old female patient came to us with complaints of eye pain since last 1 week.

Her BCVA in both eyes is 6/6 with 0.50 D sphere and near correction is N6 with +2.25 DS correction.

Her anterior segment examination is within normal limits in both eyes. Angles are wide open all round. Posterior segment showed C/D ratio 0.65 with healthy neuroretinal rim (HNRR) in right eye and C/D ratio 0.75 with thin inferior rim in left eye. Her IOPs were 21 and 24 mm Hg with CCT of 512 and 517 µm, respectively.

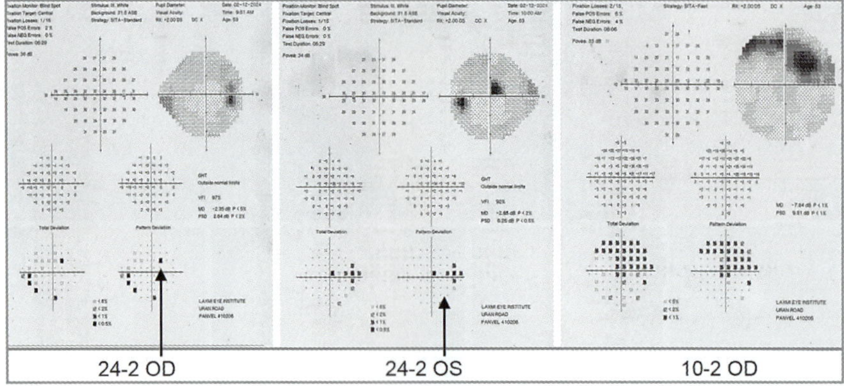

Fig. 31: Perimetry reports.

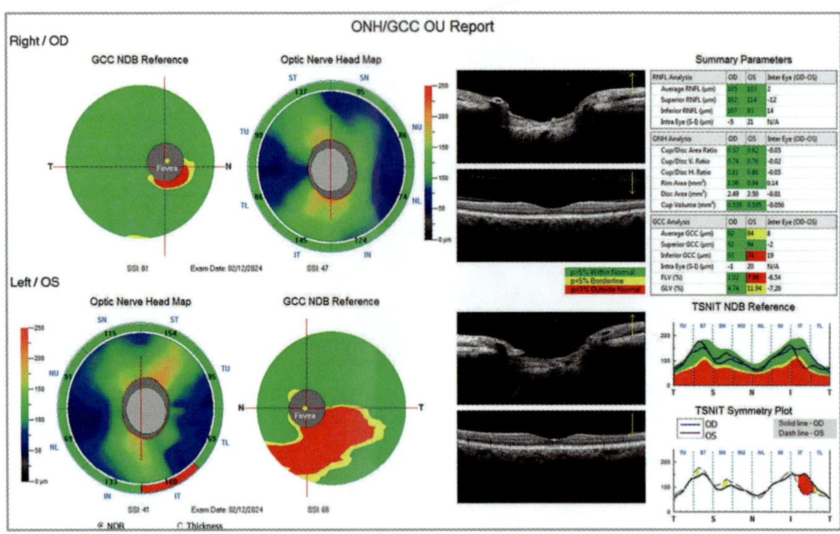

Fig. 32: Optical coherence tomography (OCT) glaucoma OU.

In the above case, even though the RE OCT looks pretty normal in the ONH, it does show a small parafoveal GCC loss in the inferior parafoveal region. In the RE, if one has a look at the perimetry in the RE, one can see a small inferior nasal step field defect and one small point showing a threshold sensitivity of $p < 0.5\%$. With glaucoma hemifield test (GHT) outside normal limits. The LE OCT clearly shows a thinning of the RNFL in the inferior temporal region, with a moderate GCC loss in the inferior quadrant more in the temporal than the nasal quadrant with focal loss volume (FLV), $p < 1\%$ and global loss volume (GLV), $p < 5\%$ **(Fig. 32)**.

Seemingly, the perimetry in the RE does not mean gross visual field defect, but if the 10-2 field of the same eye is done, the central defect is blown up to show a superior hemifield defect in the central 10°, which could mean a lot more visual functional loss in real life. Which will then lead in a relatively more aggressive treatment even for the RE.

The perimetry and OCT are tests to document functional and structural defects. There is a lot of information in both these printouts. But *one has to be a real watchdog* to look for the fine print in all that these printouts say. Interpret the report very carefully to maximize visual potential for your patient. May be just an eyeballing of the colors on these printouts, would have been losing out on the vital information that the test is providing, hence minimizing the utility of the test.

Of course, never interpret any test singly, always correlate clinically. Do the tests correlate with what you see clinically? Sometimes a totally different pathology in the area of the papillomacular bundle will mimic a glaucoma like perimetric defect like a chorioretinal patch, or a branch vein occlusion, but the fundus gives you the answer in these cases.

Looking at all this, we decided on a target of 25% decrease in IOP for BE which meant coming down to the mid-teens for the RE around 15 mm Hg and 17 mm Hg for the LE, so we decided on starting the patient with a prostaglandin which is known to result in a 30% drop in IOP. Patient is now doing well. After 6 weeks of treatment, her IOP has come down to 14 mm Hg in the RE and 16 mm Hg in the LE. Fortunately, the patient is not yet complaining of the redness of her eyes and is happy that her IOP is responding well.

Do you think this is a reliable field and can be taken as authentic/should a repeat field confirm the defects?

When will I repeat the perimetry?

How often will I repeat it? What will I look for?

Could I have instead done a SLT on this patient?

Would surgery be a treatment for this patient? If yes, When and which surgery would you advocate?

CASE 12

A 54-year-old male patient presented with a gradual loss of vision in the RE. Last refraction was done 2 years ago. Was he not a myope **(Figs. 33A and B)**?

No h/o any ocular symptoms till recently noticed diminished vision. No h/o headache, brow ache, pain around the temples, or vomiting. There was no h/o any systemic illness DM/HYT. No h/o being on any medications. No h/o intake of tobacco/alcohol. No f/h/o glaucoma.

On examination: BCVA: RE:FC= 3 m N <48, LE: 6/12 N6.

IOP: 14 and 12 mm Hg, CCT: 510 and 504 μm. AS: WNL. Pupil: Sluggish in the RE, retinal total layer (RTL) in the LE. AC: Deep and quiet in OU.

Gonioscopy: Angles open to the posterior trabecular meshwork (PTM) in OU.

Cause of diminished vision? Have a look at his fundus? Is it a central cause?

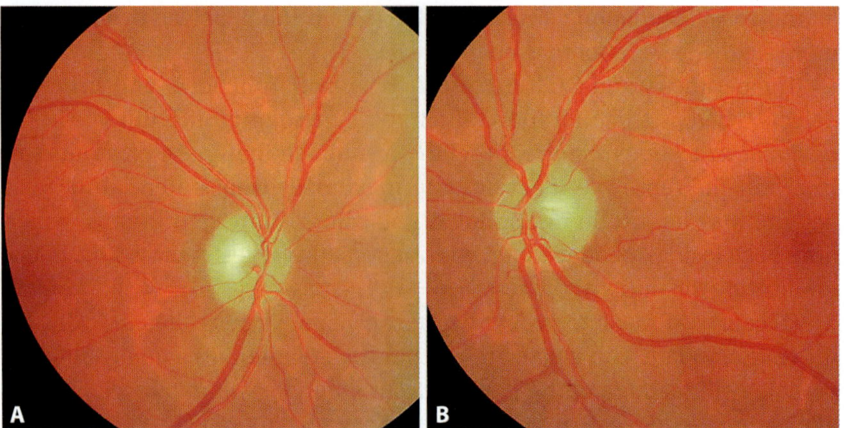

Figs. 33A and B: Show fundus pictures of the Right and the Left eye.

- Did the discs give you a clue? They look apparently OK. Is there something you are missing? Large cups? Pallor temporally in both eyes? Any diagnosis at this stage?

NTG? Why loss in one eye? Does the RE look paler than the LE? Would you want any other investigations?

We got the perimetry done. And see what we found. A bitemporal hemianopia! Some neurological pathology.

Probably near the decussation of the nasal fibers/close to the pituitary gland. What next? Referred to a neurologist/do some more investigations? An MRI was done, and a pituitary adenoma was diagnosed.

Many times, small clues like these must create curiosity to think about what next. Getting the perimetry made things very clear. The patient gave no h/o headache, vomiting to suggest a rise in the intracranial pressure. But that nasal pallor of the disc was the telltale sign. Remember that you are treating a patient and not the ocular pathology alone. No RE cataract/glaucoma. Please learn to look at the patient as a whole. Many systemic illnesses do present to us with ocular signs and symptoms. Keep your eyes and ears open. Listen well to the patient. A lot of information is provided by the patient and do not take it lightly **(Figs. 34A and B)**.

CASE 13: DR ROOPALI NERLIKAR

A 54-year-old male presented with strong f/h/o glaucoma, hypertensive on lipid lowering agents. He had been diagnosed to have POAG 9 years earlier and well controlled on travoprost HS for first 3 years. Thereafter, there was evidence of mild progression. An office diurnal showed 5 mm Hg variation between lowest and highest readings. Timolol maleate 0.5% was added in the morning and the office IOP readings were apparently stable, but he continued to show slight progression. The importance of compliance was emphasized, and option of SLT was given. He underwent the same with stabilization of

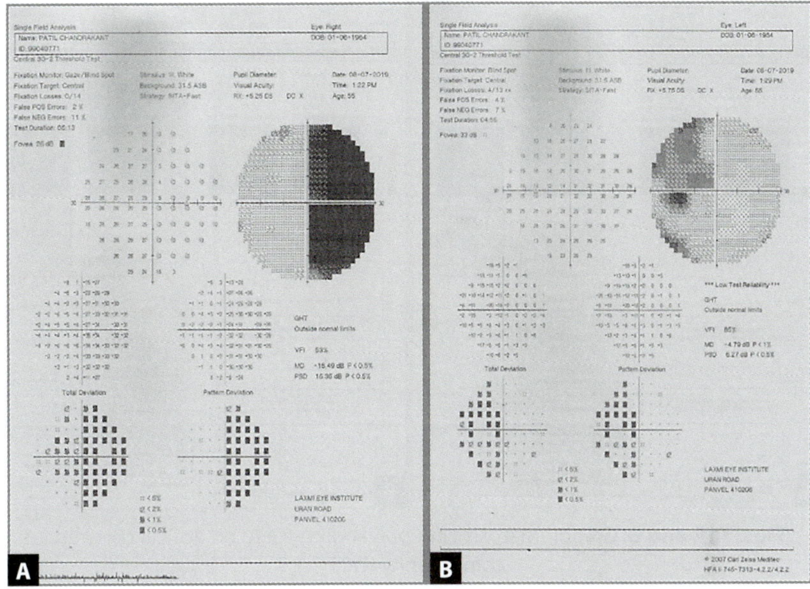

Figs. 34A and B: (A) Perimetry right eye (RE) showing temporal hemianopia; (B) Perimetry left eye (LE) showing temporal hemianopia.

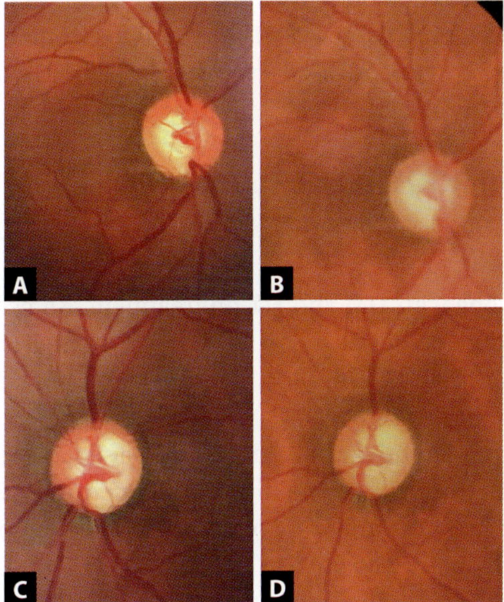

Figs. 35A to D: Fundus right and left eye.

RNFL loss on OCT and visual field loss on perimetry. Follow-up was sporadic during the pandemic and he showed further progression in his left eye, partly due to self-admitted poor compliance on the patients' part. The IOP and disease stabilized with strict adherence to medication **(Figs. 35A to D)**.

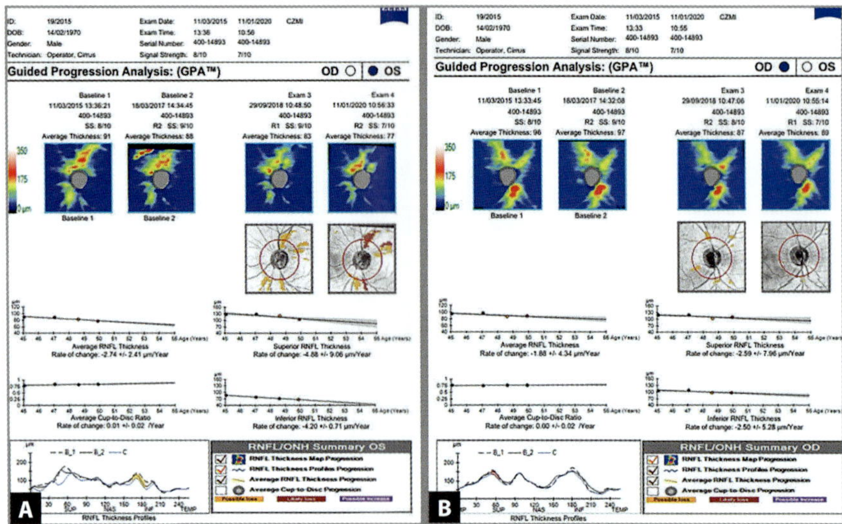

Figs. 36A and B: Granulomatosis with polyangiitis (GPA) on optical coherence tomography (OCT).

In 2024, he developed visually significant central posterior subcapsular cataract (PSC) cataract needing surgery. As he was medically well controlled with stable disease, at this point the option of left eye cataract surgery with microinvasive glaucoma surgery (MIGS) (KDB excisional goniotomy) was offered which he subsequently underwent with stable IOP off medication in that eye **(Figs. 36A and B)**.

CASE 14: DR ROOPALI NERLIKAR

An 83-year-old male presented with a known case of POAG on medical management since 12 years.

He is low myope with DM and HT on treatment, RE pseudophakic, and reported with reduction in vision.

BCVA: RE 6/12p and LE 6/18. RE good pseudophakia, LE PSC, NS 2 cataract.

Ill-sustained pupils and partial red, green color defect was noted.

IOP 32 and 36 mm Hg on maximum tolerated topical (four drugs in combination) therapy, gonioscopy open angles, and blood in Schlemm's canal noted. Pachymetry 522 and 518 μm **(Fig. 37)**.

In view of proptosis, lid retraction and chemosis, congestion of a concomitant thyroid eye disease was suspected, and he was evaluated for the same. He was found to have significant myopathy with compression of optic nerves at orbital apex on MRI orbit. He was treated with intravenous methylprednisolone followed by oral steroids and needed orbital decompression as well. Three months postsurgery, his vision had improved

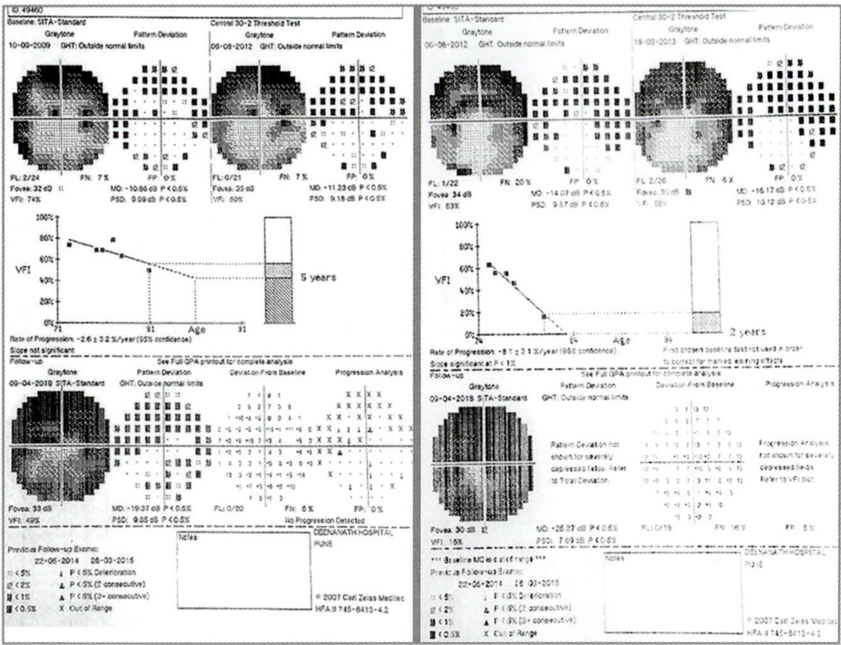

Fig. 37: Perimetry showing progression in OU.

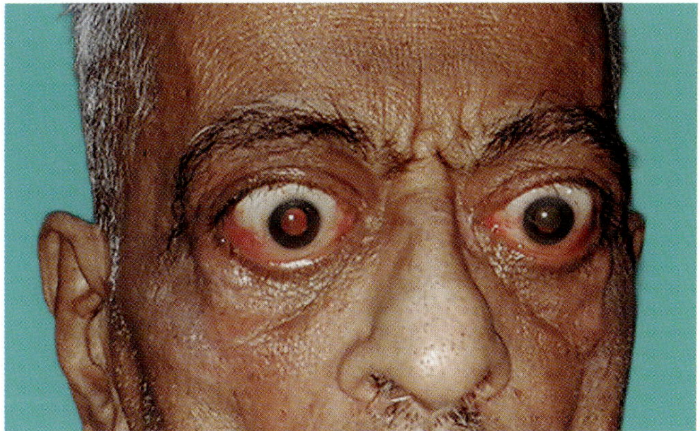

Fig. 38: Proptosis.

to 6/9 RE, 6/12 LE, color vision defects had resolved, and IOP was 16 and 20 on four medications. The field defects had improved as well. He has been given the option of combined cataract and glaucoma surgery in his left eye **(Fig. 38)**.

Index

Page numbers followed by *f* refer to figure, *fc* refer to flowchart, and *t* refer to table.

D

E

F

G